A Woman's Worth

A Woman's Worth

Health, Stigma and Discrimination in India

SOPHIE COUSINS

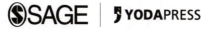

Los Angeles | London | New Delhi
Singapore | Washington DC | Melbourne

First published in 2020 by

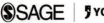

SAGE Publications India Pvt Ltd
B1/I-1 Mohan Cooperative Industrial Area
Mathura Road, New Delhi 110 044, India
www.sagepub.in

SAGE Publications Inc
2455 Teller Road
Thousand Oaks, California 91320, USA

SAGE Publications Ltd
1 Oliver's Yard, 55 City Road
London EC1Y 1SP, United Kingdom

SAGE Publications Asia-Pacific Pte Ltd
18 Cross Street #10-10/11/12
China Square Central
Singapore 048423

YODA Press
79 Gulmohar Enclave
New Delhi 110049
www.yodapress.co.in

Published by Vivek Mehra for SAGE Publications India Pvt Ltd. Typeset in 10.5/13pt Adobe Caslon Pro by Fidus Design Pvt Ltd, Chandigarh.

Library of Congress Cataloging-in-Publication Data Available

ISBN: 978-93-5328-976-8 (HB)

SAGE Yoda Team: Arpita Das, Ishita Gupta, Amrita Dutta and Sandhya Gola

To the women who let me into their homes and their lives.
And to my Mum, the woman I look most up to in life.

Thank you for choosing a SAGE product!
If you have any comment, observation or feedback,
I would like to personally hear from you.

Please write to me at **contactceo@sagepub.in**

Vivek Mehra, Managing Director and CEO, SAGE India.

Bulk Sales

SAGE India offers special discounts
for purchase of books in bulk.
We also make available special imprints
and excerpts from our books on demand.

For orders and enquiries, write to us at

Marketing Department
SAGE Publications India Pvt Ltd
B1/I-1, Mohan Cooperative Industrial Area
Mathura Road, Post Bag 7
New Delhi 110044, India

E-mail us at **marketing@sagepub.in**

Subscribe to our mailing list
Write to **marketing@sagepub.in**

This book is also available as an e-book.

Ai Maon, behnon, beityon duniya ki zeenat tumsay hai
Mulkon ki basti ho tum hi, qaumon ki izzat tumsay hai

O Sisters, mothers, daughters
You are the ornaments of the world
You are the life of the nations
The dignity of civilisations

Altaf Hussain Hali

Contents

Author's Note

This book is the accumulation of stories I have gathered over the last four years. It is a work of non-fiction that is backed up by extensive research, countless field visits and numerous interviews with experts. Some of the stories in this book were first published by different media publications including the *Guardian*, the *Caravan*, *Mosaic Science* and *Elle*.

For stylistic reasons, some chapters are dated, others are not. Some names of people have been changed as per their request. Lastly, currency conversions from Indian Rupees to US Dollars were made as of 22 August 2019.

Acknowledgements

There are so many people I need to thank, for without their knowledge, support, love, hospitality and encouragement, this book would not have been possible. I truly see this book as a collective effort of all the people who have helped me over the years and there are too many to name.

In no particular order I want to thank my publisher, Arpita Das, for taking a chance on me. I am full of immense gratitude to her for giving me the creative freedom to pursue this book.

To Sutapa Neogi, Vinoj Manning, Poonam Muttreja, Mridu Gupta, Jashodhara Dasgupta and Arun Kumar, thank you for your patience, for answering my endless questions, and for facilitating so many of my trips across India.

To my dearest friends Anant Asthana, Gautam Basu, Snigdha Basu and Vidya Krishnan, thank you for teaching me so much about your country. To Amrita Nandy, thank you for your expert translation. I will always cherish the time we spent travelling across India together. Thank you to Annabel Symington, for our time together in Kathmandu. You made that city a better place.

There are far too many to name but to all the activists, strangers and local reporters who went out of their way to help me with my work—from translating, to connecting me with your sources, to providing a bed to rest my head on at night, thank you.

To Alison Francis, Claire Rogers, Nicole Amdur and Katie Huber, thank you for always being there for me. I will be forever grateful for our late night chats and endless glasses of wine, and above all, our life-long friendship.

And to Martin. Thank you for understanding my love of India and for understanding that this was something I needed to do.

To Pete, thank you for our entertaining table tennis breaks on long, hard days. That time away from the computer helped me to clear my head and overcome writer's block. Thank you to my sister, Maddie, for your visits always invigorated me.

To my parents, thank you for your endless support and love. Thank you for always encouraging me to follow my dreams, no matter how much it has made you both worry.

And lastly, to the women of India who let me into their homes and their hearts. I wish you all the happiness and strength in the world.

Preface

When I arrived in India as a backpacker almost a decade ago, I had no idea what the country had in store for me. For as long as I could remember, I had always dreamed of visiting this enchanting, far away place. I was gifted an Indian cookbook one year for Christmas and for days on end I poured over the photos of the sweeping tea gardens of Assam, the Buddhist monasteries of Ladakh, and the backwaters of Kerala. I was fascinated by this country that offered so much and the recipes—while they never tasted anything like the food I've eaten in India—nevertheless instilled more of a desire to visit.

When I landed in New Delhi early one May morning I was overwhelmed. The people, the smells, the sounds, the sights. It was a true overload of the senses. Despite being told May was the hottest month to visit, being an Australian I thought India's heat would be nothing compared with what we went through every summer. How very wrong I was.

While my relationship with India initially began as an intense love/hate one, it has developed into one of deep love, admiration and respect.

This book is the accumulation of several years spent in India, travelling to some of the most far-flung places. It is predominantly focused on the north—a part of the country I have always been most fascinated with.

It took me four years to collect and write the stories in this book. I worked largely on a shoe-string budget, relying often on strangers' and friends' overwhelming generosity. From being housed in the remote villages of Jharkhand, to being driven by motorbike through the forests of Assam, to being fed dal and chapatti in Uttar Pradesh, I will be forever grateful.

To this end, I see this book as a collective effort of all the people who have helped me over the years.

This book is split into eight chapters with each chapter focusing on a specific women's health issue. It is chronologically ordered to demonstrate how gender inequality, stigma and discrimination affect women throughout their life course. I of course could not include every health issue that plagues women. For want of not prolonging the book unnecessarily, I picked the issues that I felt warranted an in-depth look, and the ones that I believe could contribute most to ongoing discussions.

You cannot generalise such a diverse country like India, home to more than 1.3 billion people. It would be wrong. And by no means do I want the individual stories here to come across as making sweeping generalisations about women and India.

The women's stories I have selected to tell are, however, powerful in themselves and from my limited attempt I do hope they present a true picture of the situation. As an outsider I have tried to understand the situation for women here to my best ability.

It is only fitting that I finish writing this book at the very place I began writing my first journal on my first trip here all those years ago: McLeod Ganj, the home of His Holiness, the Dalai Lama, overlooking the Himalayas.

I hope that this book will add something to the literature available on the health of women in India.

Sophie Cousins
31 March 2019

Part I

The Struggle to Survive

CHAPTER 1

Sex Selection
Desperate Measures for a Son

The road from India's chaotic capital, New Delhi, to a village in the neighbouring state of Haryana is a sad glimpse into the future of India's urban landscape. On the border of the two states stand ghastly towering apartment blocks that have been carefully positioned amid desolate land and daily labourers completing arduous work. The blocks are built on the promise of the 'dream'—luxury affordable western living just a stone's throw away from the businesses, bars and restaurants of Gurgaon (also known as Gurugram), one of Delhi's satellite cities also known for its stifling pollution. The apartment blocks—which look incongruous compared to their surroundings—are not only a reminder of the great and increasing divide between the rich and poor but also signify how urbanisation and globalisation is rapidly transforming India, and how so many are being left behind.

It's October 2016 and I'm travelling to meet Meena, a then 23-year-old woman who lives with her husband and in-laws in Sampla, a village in the south-east district of Rohtak in Haryana. The state is one of India's wealthiest with its burgeoning city of Gurgaon, along with its major agricultural, dairy farming and manufacturing industries. The vast majority of the land is arable and almost all of it is cultivated, providing a rich source of work for daily labourers.

The road into Sampla is unpaved and pot-holed. In the monsoon season—which I experience at a later visit—the soccer-ball-sized pot-holes fill up and partially engulf the village. There's no drainage in sight. Sampla is a maze of narrow alleyways comprised of mud-brick homes with colourful front doors, cow and buffalo sheds and barefoot children playing hopscotch.

Meena is wearing a dark purple dress and a thin red and blue dupatta scarf which she drapes over her slim face. Her two-and-a-half-year-old daughter hangs off her shoulder as she sits on a small wooden step to make chai. Her home is sparse, with a single charpoy—an Indian-style bed made of rope—positioned in the back of the one-room home.

Meena's husband is a daily labourer who is out tending the fields. Meena is a housewife who spends her day cleaning their home, cooking and looking after their daughter. When she's not busy, she often passes her time by listening to her three sisters-in-law and mother-in-law gossip.

She doesn't contribute much to the conversations, though. In fact, Meena's unease with her family-in-law is palpable. She doesn't lift her gaze from the floor when she speaks or when she is spoken to. It's as if she's been relegated to the bottom of the family hierarchy, where her in-laws are waiting for her to do something wrong, like not put enough sugar in their chai.

In February 2016, Meena expected to give birth to a healthy baby. She and her husband were expecting their second child would be a boy. But their lives were upended when Meena had a stillbirth at a nearby hospital.[1]

'The doctor told me the child died in my womb. He said there was no heart beat. There was no explanation,' she says.

Six months earlier, while Meena was in her first trimester, she had consumed what are known as sex-selection drugs (SSDs)—traditional

---

[1] Part of this story has been published previously in Sophie Cousins, India's war on the sex selection drugs linked to stillbirths, *The Guardian*, 27 October 2016. Available at: https://www.theguardian.com/global-development/2016/oct/27/india-war-sex-selection-drugs-linked-to-stillbirths-haryana-pregnant-women

remedies that Indian women turn to, or are forced to turn to—in their and their families' desire to have sons.

But what most women don't realise is that the sex of a child cannot be changed in the womb; that they are being scammed.

'I took the drugs because we wanted a male child—because my first baby was female. I vomited a lot after it. I couldn't digest it,' Meena says.

The drugs are typically taken six to 10 weeks after conception and they are sold to women through an underground network involving cycle rickshaw drivers and midwives, who connect families to sellers who are often local quacks. They cost between ₹200 and ₹3500 (US$3–$50) and women are promised a male child if they take the drugs—which come in powder or tablet form—following a very strict ritual.

Meena was ordered to take the drugs early one Monday morning just after the moon had given way to the rising red sun with a fresh glass of cow's milk while looking at her husband. After consuming the milk she had to chant a series of prayers, asking for a son.

She went through her pregnancy believing she would soon give birth to a boy, which she knew was critical to appeasing her husband and his family. And by doing so, Meena would have fulfilled her primary role as a woman in Indian society: to produce a son.

But little did Meena know that the drugs often contain phytoestrogens —compounds from plants that are similar to the female sex hormone oestrogen—in levels beyond what is considered safe. Phytoestrogens, as well as heavy metals—which have also been found in the drugs—are linked to birth defects and stillbirths. In fact, research led by the Public Health Foundation of India, an autonomous foundation based in New Delhi, has found that SSDs are a factor in 20 per cent of all stillbirths in Haryana (Neogi et al., 2015).

It's estimated that up to 60 per cent of women in Haryana who have one daughter take SSDs for their second birth (S. Neogi, personal communication). It's a figure that has led researchers to wonder how many of the estimated 592,100 stillbirths in India every year—the highest number in the world—are a direct consequence of SSDs.

But Meena didn't know this when she took the drugs. She just knew she had to produce a son or there would be consequences.

In October 2016, eight months on from her stillbirth and when I meet her for the first time, she's in absolute denial that the drugs she consumed could have been responsible for her stillbirth. Her family say it's impossible that 'traditional' remedies could have caused her any harm.

Her reaction is no surprise—the quack who gave her the drugs says it's Meena's fault she had a stillbirth. She must not have followed the ritual properly, he told her.

Instead of being given ample time to mourn the loss of her child, the pressure is on for Meena to try again for a son.

'I would like to take a gap [but] my husband is insisting on having another child. I don't know. We'll try again for another male baby,' she tells me.

Before I leave her home, she lifts her head cautiously, gazing around so no one else can see. Our eyes—hers, which are slightly visible through her thin dupatta—meet for the first time. She whispers in Hindi, 'If I take the drugs again, will it be harmful?'

✳

Stigma and discrimination against women in India begins before birth. And there is no greater evidence of the unequal and subordinate status of women in Indian society than the practice of sex selection.

Parents' desire for sons is so prevalent that sex-selective abortion and female foeticide—abortion of female foetuses by illegal means—has given India one of the world's most skewed sex ratios. According to the most recent Census in 2011, there were 914 girls to every 1,000 boys for children up to the age of six (Office of the Registrar General and Census Commissioner, 2011). In some north Indian states like Haryana—where the preference for boys is strongest—that ratio dropped to 830.

There are dire predictions that the ratio is going to decline even further, with calculations it will drop to a national level of 898 girls to every 1,000 boys by 2031 (Ministry of Statistics and Programme Implementation, 2017).

According to the government's 2017–18 annual economic survey, this entrenched preference for boys has resulted in more than 63 million women 'missing' across India (Ministry of Finance, 2018, p.105). In other words, India has 63 million fewer women that it should have. That is roughly the population of the United Kingdom. Missing.

The survey also found that more than two million women go missing across age groups every year due to sex-selective abortion, disease, neglect, or inadequate nutrition (Ministry of Finance, 2018, p.112). (The neglect of girls, and the favouring of boys for nutritious food and medical care is a topic that is discussed at length in the subsequent chapter.)

So why is there a preference for sons in Indian society?

The ingrained preference for male offspring stretches back centuries and is motivated by a complex web of social, economic, religious and cultural factors.

The first Indian census in 1872 showed evidence of this preference through the marked gap between the number of boys and girls, men and women—a trend which has continued to manifest to the present day. In a deeply patriarchal society—a society which continues to reinforce male favourability through a vicious cycle of gender discrimination—girls are considered a liability rather than an asset.

Parents expect sons to provide financially for the family, while daughters are seen as a burden because they drain finances through dowries. A dowry is paid in the form of cash and goods such as jewellery and household appliances to the groom or his parents by the bride's family. While the practice was outlawed in 1961, it's a custom that stubbornly resists change and reform, and one that places monumental financial burdens on the bride's family.

Daughters are married away into other households where they become the sole responsibility of another family. Sons, meanwhile, are considered as the only ones able to continue family lineage and care for parents as they age. In a patrilineal society, property and inheritance is passed on to sons who are also seen as vital to defend or exercise the family's power and to perform important religious duties.

The system, as it stands today, rewards the birth of a son, and penalises the birth of a daughter.

'At the end of the day, boys are simply valued more than girls, and the rest is just a justification for that,' Anita Raj, director of the Centre on Gender Equity and Health at the University of California, San Diego, tells me.

✳

The 1980s saw the proliferation of sex screening technologies, primarily the ultrasound machine. The cheap technology, used in the developed world in the context of pregnancy to evaluate the health of the foetus, became almost exclusively used in India to determine the gender of an unborn child.

It wasn't the first technology to come to India which could determine the sex of a foetus. Amniocentesis, a method used to detect foetal anomalies by removing amniotic fluid from the sac surrounding the foetus, became available in the 1970s. It too could determine the sex of a foetus and its use corresponded with the legalisation of abortion up to 20 weeks under the Medical Termination of Pregnancy (MTP) Act, 1971.

In those early years, access to amniocentesis was limited, largely because of its prohibitive cost. But what did become immediately clear was that any technology that could determine the sex of a foetus would be used for female foeticide.

The liberalisation of India's economy from the late 1980s enabled agreements between national and global markets which facilitated the import or production of ultrasound machines.

Cashing in on the opportunity, doctors imported the machines from across the globe to make sex determination—even in far-flung rural areas—not only accessible and popular but to a large extent, expected. The ultrasound machine legitimised society's preference for boys over girls, and in doing so fuelled a fast-declining sex ratio.

A December 1991 newspaper article in the *New York Times* from Rohtak, Haryana—the district where Meena lives—details just how blatantly the ultrasound was responsible for skewing India's sex ratio (Gargan). The article highlights how acceptable finding out the sex of an unborn child had become—and thus choosing which ones to keep—by zooming in on a sign hanging up at a local clinic which read, 'Ultrasound. Healthy Boy or Girl' (1991). The word 'healthy', the article notes, is painted so meticulously that the sign appears to read, 'Boy or Girl'.

'If the test says girl, then she will have an abortion,' Jagmati Sangwan, Haryana's then-state branch leader of the All India Democratic Women's Association, told the newspaper (Gargan, 1991).

'We want to make these sex determination tests illegal. We think it is an attack on the existence of women.'

In 1994, under pressure from activists including Sangwan, the central government outlawed the use of ultrasound machines to determine the sex of a foetus. It limited the use of prenatal diagnosis to a list of selected congenital conditions and established a bureaucracy to regulate the sale of ultrasound machines.

But despite the ban, the law remained wilfully unenforced. Eventually the Supreme Court of India was forced to intervene in 2003. The Court issued directives to state governments across the country demanding they raise awareness about the law and increase surveillance of clinics providing ultrasounds. The court also advised the central government to amend the law.

In 2004 the law was amended to become the Pre-Conception and Pre-Natal Diagnostic Techniques (PCPNDT) Act to not only deter and punish prenatal sex screening and female foeticide but to also ban preconception sex-selection techniques such as sperm sorting—a technique where a sperm cell is specifically chosen because of its sex chromosome. The law had finally moved to ban all forms of sex selection.

Today, clinics and hospitals across India have replaced the 'Ultrasound. Healthy Boy or Girl' sign with one that reads, 'Here pre-natal sex determination (boy or girl before birth) is not done, it is a punishable act'.

But a sign and a threat of punishment is not enough to deter families. At the end of the day the desire to have a son will persist, at least until the root cause of this desire is addressed. And as long as demand for such technology continues unabated, there is no shortage of doctors willing to break the law.

'The ultrasound was India's biggest curse. A doctor wants money and a woman wants to know the sex of her child—it's a mutual benefit and both keep their mouths shut,' Varun Arora, a doctor who works at the Post Graduate Institute of Medical Sciences in Rohtak, Haryana, says.

'The demand in society for a male child is so high that even if the laws and acts are implemented, people will find a way.'

❋

In early 2015, Prime Minister Narendra Modi's government launched a national campaign, Beti Bachao, Beti Padhao (Educate the Girl Child, Save the Girl Child), with renewed focus on enforcing the law that forbids sex-selective abortion and diagnostic techniques that are used for female foeticide, along with promoting girls' education.

But by the government's own admission on the campaign's website, executing the PCPNDT Act 'suffers from the bottlenecks of implementation, and there have been few convictions so far. The major difficulty relates to proving that an offence has occurred, since it takes place behind closed doors, with connivance between the medical service provider and parents' (Ministry of Women and Child Development, 2015).

A fundamental problem with relying on the PCPNDT Act to curb sex selection is that it oversimplifies a highly complex problem by placing the onus on doctors rather than society.

Moreover, as ultrasounds are routinely used in maternal care, detecting all acts that take place secretly and illegally is impossible.

Relying on a law—one that is, at best, occasionally enforced—neglects to ask the question: why are boys more valued in society than girls? How can this mindset be changed?

It would be remiss to ignore that the Educate the Girl Child, Save the Girl Child campaign is a step forward in the right direction in that it at least recognises the importance of promoting girls' education and by doing so fuels a public discourse on the matter.

But the campaign fundamentally fails to recognise that sex selection cannot be seen as an isolated phenomenon among parents who do not educate their girls or see the value in it. In fact, demand for a son among the educated, urban, middle and upper-class is greater than those in rural areas who are less likely to educate their girls for many reasons but primarily poverty (Pande and Malhotra, 2006). Gender discrimination itself does not discriminate.

Awareness about the illegality of sex determination is greater among the educated, many of whom can afford to by-pass the law and look for solutions outside of India.

In recent years Thailand has emerged as a popular destination for Indian couples who want to secure a prized baby boy. Using Preimplantation Genetic Diagnosis (PGD)—a reproductive technology which helps select the best embryos to prevent genetic diseases from being passed on to the child—along with In vitro fertilisation (IVF), enables couples to legally choose their baby's sex.

Various news reports have detailed how common the procedure is among Indians flocking to Thailand. It's become such a trend that it has been labelled 'Bangkok Boys'—baby boys conceived during holidays in the chaotic capital.

A 2010 newspaper report in a daily Indian newspaper, *Hindustan Times* quotes a major Bangkok hospital spokesperson who tells the journalist, 'A lot of Indians come to our hospital for IVF for sex selection … there's been a drastic increase in the last two years' (Sharma).

Needless to say, most Indians do not have US$10,000 to spare to fly to Bangkok and undergo IVF and PGD. But there are new and cheaper methods of sex detection available on the global market including a blood test at seven weeks of gestation which can reliably predict the sex of a child. As medical technology continues to evolve, ways to determine the sex of a foetus will only become easier and more affordable. This will inevitably raise fundamental problems and questions for India's policy and law-makers who will need to decide what can be regulated and what—like air travel—cannot.

Recognising this, in 2017 the Indian Supreme Court ordered Google and other search engines to censor online advertisements for sex detection tests which had infiltrated the internet. Unearthing where to get sex determination test done had simply become a matter of a click of a button.

✳

While the law prohibiting sex selection has failed to do what it was meant to do, for all its shortfalls, it has given well-meaning doctors impetus to disrupt the cycle of structural violence against women by refusing to participate in female foeticide. By doing so, they have drawn attention to the grave problem. There are countless doctors who are committed to stopping sex selection and actively campaign against it.

Dr Ganesh Rakh, a doctor from Pune, a sprawling city in the western Indian state of Maharashtra, is a prime example. In 2007 he opened a small hospital in his home town but quickly became overwhelmed by an event that would play out on a daily basis: celebration and joy when he would deliver a boy; tears of disappointment and sorrow when he would deliver a girl.

'The biggest challenge for a doctor is to tell relatives that a patient has died. For me, it was equally difficult to tell families that they'd had a daughter,' he says.

In 2012 he decided to do something. He launched a campaign, Mulgi Vachva Abhiyan (Campaign to Save the Girl Child), in which he began delivering baby girls free of charge. It was his attempt at altering society's attitudes towards girls, a simple yet generous decision that he continues to do today. He also decided that since a boy's birth was so jovially celebrated by the family, the hospital would also celebrate the birth of a girl with sweets and cake. The only tears he wants in the newborn unit is tears of joy. Dr Rakh's work has inspired more than 17,000 other Indian doctors to follow in his footsteps by pledging to reduce fees, or charge nothing at all when delivering baby girls.

But the harsh reality is that for all the laudable doctors like Dr Rakh who celebrate the birth of a girl child, there will inevitably always be the doctors who, for the right price, will continue to perform ultrasounds and female foeticide.

✳

Many Indians are unaware that a law prohibiting sex selection exists. Many don't need to know because they simply don't care if they have girls or boys, or both. This is particularly true in southern states like Kerala, which has the highest sex ratio in India with 1084 females per 1000 males, according to the most recent census (Office of the Registrar General and Census Commissioner, 2011).

Many more are cognisant that the law exists but do not take any threat of persecution seriously.

In 2008, more than a decade after the initial law against sex selection had been implemented, Haryana became the first state to reach five convictions under the PCPNDT Act.

In recent years, however, states including Haryana and Punjab—the two states with the country's most skewed sex ratio—have publicly cracked down on doctors performing illegal ultrasounds. Hundreds of complaints against doctors have been lodged, but again, there have only been a handful of convictions. Government officials in Haryana I spoke with admitted that offenders too often get bail and are back in business within a few months.

The raids and arrests—which are meant to further deter doctors and families through social media and news coverage—enable other willing doctors to charge more for the procedure. This often results in families taking loans from unscrupulous moneylenders and travelling as far as 300 km to find out the sex of their baby. But for those who do not have the means to pay exorbitant prices for an ultrasound and drive across state lines, it just means they will look for easier and cheaper options. And this is where sex selection drugs (SSDs) come in.

✳

India is a country with a thriving informal healthcare system, one that is heavily reliant on traditional medicine from local faith healers, to bone setters and Ayurvedic medicines.

Much of it is harmless and, as many believe, helpful for minor ailments. What is harmful though is that millions of people across India put their lives in the hands of quacks who promise to cure cancer or to even deliver them a son.

The reliance on medicine outside the confines of a hospital's walls is not only steeped in history and tradition but has also continued to thrive because of the systemic failings of the formal healthcare system.

Sex selection drugs are sold on the pretext that they are indigenous medicines and therefore safe no matter how large the dose. But SSDs contain phytoestrogens, as well as heavy metals which are linked to birth defects and stillbirths. They also contain soy products, food additives and other plant steroids. They are given in varied doses and doled out by faith healers, quacks, grocers, doctors and even rickshaw drivers who are also in on the racket.

'I was shocked and surprised at what the samples contained,' Dr Abhijit Ganguli, a biotechnology expert who analysed dozens of SSD samples from Haryana, tells me.

'It's unnatural for anyone to take these drugs for any period of time.'

In addition to being at high risk of having a stillbirth, research shows that pregnant women who consume the drugs are almost three times more likely to give birth to a baby with visible birth defects (Neogi et al., 2017). Across north India, the likelihood that a woman will use the drugs—or be forced to use them—is heavily dependent on the number of girl children she has already had. Birth order is a significant determinant for sex selection.

Research suggests that about 10 per cent of pregnant women with one girl child across north India consume SSDs in their attempt to secure a son; this figure increases to 40 per cent if a woman already has two daughters (Manchanda et al., 2011).

Despite the shocking figures which illustrate how rampant the use of SSDs is, officials I spoke with in Haryana are adamant that law enforcement, rather than working to change people's perception of girls, is the way to tackle the issue.

'Nothing can be done to change people's mindset. Nobody wants a girl child. A woman is only respected as a wife if she bears a male child. Only law enforcement will work to save as many girl children as possible,' says Dr Arora from the Post Graduate Institute of Medical Sciences in Rohtak, Haryana.

✳

In July 2018 I travel to Behlba, a village in the Rohtak district of Haryana. Like Sampla village, the road into Behlba is jarring and pot-holed. It's the height of the monsoon season and the village is partially submerged after a recent downpour. The streets and laneways are thick with mud and floating trash. Wearing shorts and singlets, young boys make the most of a lack of drainage by jumping off buildings' into the streets which look like a polluted brown lagoon.

I enter the aqua blue two-room house to a beaming Meena who greets me at the door. It's been a while since we last met.

Her presence is striking. She is confident and garrulous. She no longer wears a dupatta swept across her face nor does she stare at the floor when she speaks or when she is spoken to. She offers an explanation for her change before I get the opportunity to ask.

'I have this feeling of freedom here away from my family-in-law,' she says.

This is her parents' home.

Something else has changed in Meena's life, which is another source of her contentment: she has had a son.

Meena, now 25-years-old, runs to the kitchen where her sister is looking after one-year-old Manish. She carries him, hanging off her right hip, through a small cobblestoned yard and back to the main bedroom where her family members have gathered. Manish is wearing a white singlet and thick eyeliner to ward off the evil eye. His few strands of black hair have been neatly oiled to the side. He's passed around from uncle to aunty to grandma, until he finally rests on the knees of Meena's father who bobs him up and down, stirring a giggle from everyone in the room.

'I feel very good. I was so happy to have a son. No more children now. I'm finished,' Meena says.

After her stillbirth in 2016, Meena resisted pressure from her husband and mother-in-law to take sex selection drugs again. No matter how much time passed, the pain of losing a baby was raw. She didn't want to risk losing another child.

'I didn't take the drugs this time because I found out that it's not good for the baby's health,' she tells me, referring to a conversation I had previously been privy to between her and researchers from the Public Health Foundation of India.

Despite Meena's resolve not to take drugs for her third pregnancy, the reality is that had she had a girl, she would have had to continue trying for a boy. She didn't know what she'd be forced to do to get the necessary result, but it's likely she would have had to take the drugs again.

'If Manish would have been a girl, I would have had to continue to try for a boy because you know, in a village it's mandatory to have a boy,' she says.

I ask Meena why a boy is necessary—why she believes that boys are more valuable than girls. Her response is symbolic of the way in which girls in India are brought up: they are led to believe they are inferior and the only way to improve their status within their family and society is to have a son.

'Only a boy will take our family name to the [next] generation and earn money and take care of the family. A girl usually gets married and goes to another house. Obviously it's important for a girl to study but only after she's married and moved to her in-laws,' she tells me.

✳

For decades the Indian government has been on a mission to control population growth. The proliferation of family planning has meant that more and more women have had the opportunity to control when and if to have children, and how many.

In the last three decades, fertility rates have almost halved from 4.5 in 1985 to 2.3 in 2016 according to the World Bank (2018). This decrease is a result of myriad factors including increased access to family planning and education, increased socio-economic status and urbanisation.

But as fertility levels across the country have fallen sharply and a small family has become the desired norm—particularly among those who live in cities—so has the desire for an ideal sex composition of children.

Too often the poor and uneducated are blamed for India's skewed sex ratio. Time and again the argument goes that with economic development and modernity, this entrenched preference for a son will dissipate.

One doesn't have to look far to see this inherent blame playing out in government policies. One prime example is the doling out of cash to women when they give birth to daughters, an initiative which some states began in 2007. The payment scheme, which is designed to discourage women from aborting female foetuses, only stands to change the behaviour of the poor. The scheme's goal is for daughters to be seen as an asset rather than a liability but in doing so it simultaneously recognises the extent to which the dowry system still operates.

Another example, as previously discussed, is the Save a Girl Child, Educate a Girl Child campaign which focuses on promoting girls' education as a means to overcoming sex selection and gender discrimination.

The importance of girls' education cannot be overestimated. But a fundamental shortfall of the Save the Girl Child, Educate a Girl Child campaign is that while advocating for girls' education, it fails to actually address what takes girls out of school: society's obsession with marriage.

Another element of the campaign is the Sukanya Samriddhi Account, (Girl Child Prosperity Account) which is a saving scheme targeted at the parents of girl children. The scheme encourages parents to build a fund for the future education and marriage expenses for their female child. The fund provides an interest rate of more than eight per cent to those who sign up.

Of course having a saving scheme for a child's future is a smart investment. But again, this specific scheme only stands to change the behaviour of the poor. And by signalling out marriage as a major expense—and one that must be saved for—again implies that the dowry system is alive and well.

The determinants of sex selection are a complex web of factors including birth order, desire to limit family size, increased socio-economic status and urbanisation, son preference and the low value of daughters in society, education, and the availability of and access to illegal sex determination technologies.

Research shows that women with higher education and who are from a higher socio-economic status are more likely to resort to sex determination and female foeticide than their less educated counterparts (Pande and Malhotra, 2006). This is further confirmed by the breakdown in sex ratios across India's states and territories which reveal that sex selection is more popular among the wealthier states, such as Haryana.

Why is this the case? Quite simply, women with higher education and who are from families with a higher disposable income have more knowledge and resources to access the required technology. They also have lower fertility, and with lower fertility comes the greater desire to control the sex of the offspring. Recent research by the World Bank found that Indian women with eight or more years of education in urban and rural areas are the main users of sex-selective abortion (Portner, 2015).

Research like this is critical because it highlights that despite laws and policies which promote gender equality and prohibit sex selection, deep-seated norms, traditions and values will prevail. And in the context of increasing urbanisation, one can only expect that as more people want smaller families, a preference for sons will continue to thrive.

✳

The systematic abuse of girls and women—millions of whom don't even get to see the light of day—has resulted in an oversupply of men. According to the latest Census, India has an excess of 37 million males (Office of the Registrar General and Census Commissioner, 2011).

A report on women's agency and child rights by India's Planning Commission said the consequences of a declining child sex ratio was a 'silent demographic disaster in the making', which will have adverse implications for women including increased trafficking for sexual exploitation, 'bought' brides, rape and violence (2011, p. 28).

In a culture that is deeply obsessed with marriage, one demographer estimates that if current levels of sex selection persist, by 2065, 10 per cent of Indian men will be single at age 50 (Guilmoto, 2012, p.77).

The implications are grave.

Decades of sex selection has already created a surplus of bachelors in states where sex selection has been most rife: Haryana and Punjab.

This surplus of bachelors means that men have to look outside their villages, towns and cities for women to marry. For India's most vulnerable girls and young women, this only exacerbates their risk of being trafficked—not only to become brides, but also domestic servants and often sex workers.

A recent assessment report on human trafficking in India found with Haryana and Punjab's deeply skewed sex ratio, 'it is impossible to find a bride for each man, and "importing a bride" has become the only solution' (United Nations Office on Drugs and Crime, 2013, p. 10).

Every year thousands of girls and young women are trafficked by one means or another to north India where they are exploited, treated like a slave and face the risk of sexual and physical violence. Some are lured by imposters who trawl impoverished villages proclaiming their love for different girls; others are kidnapped. Most of the bride-trafficked women and girls come from poor villages in India's north-east including West Bengal, Bihar and Assam.

Teenager Almima will never forget 15 March 2016, the day she waved goodbye to her parents as she jumped on board a bus with her sister.

She believed the pair were visiting a city not far from their village for a few days.

The girls, who are from Assam, a state famous for its sprawling tea plantations, were travelling to Barpeta, a city in the western region. Almima was excited; it was the first time she'd left her village which sits on the banks of the Brahmaputra River.

Once they reached Barpeta, there was a man called Salim waiting for them. Salim told the girls to get on a train to New Delhi, almost 2,000 km away. Almima followed her older sister's instructions: do what he says and get on the train.

Little did Almima know that she was being trafficked and that her sister was married to Salim. After arriving in Delhi, her sister left her with Salim and his network of traffickers.

She was soon transported across the border to Haryana.

'I had never left my village. I was studying. I would never have left,' she tells me, wiping her delicate tears off her face with her bright pink scarf.

Almima had been sold for ₹60,000 (US$850) to a wealthy family which included three older men. She knew the family was wealthy because they had a big house made of bricks—a stark contrast to the mud-hut she lived in.

Overnight she became a wife—to any of the men in the home—and a domestic slave.

'When I heard I'd been sold, I tried to escape but the men would torture me. They would punch me when I told them I wanted to go home. They locked me inside a room at night,' she says.

'I had to escape from that place or I would have died.'

Almima's escape reads like a movie script.

A few weeks into her ordeal, she found a mobile phone on the bed of one of the men's sisters when the family was out. She secretly called her family who was eventually able to send help.

When Almima's parents brought her back to their village, news had spread about her traumatic experience.

She was labelled a prostitute and a dirty sex slave. She was deemed unmarriageable.

'People here are not good. They tell me I'm a sex slave and that I'm a prostitute. They still say rubbish about me,' she says.

She hasn't seen her sister since arriving home—she thinks she's with Salim in Delhi still.

She did, however, call her. 'I called my sister and asked: why did you do this to me?'

Her sister hung up.

✳

What about the men, a majority of whom do not buy brides, but cannot find a wife? What will come of these surplus men?

A contentious 2002 study, A Surplus of Men, A Deficit of Peace: Security and Sex Ratios in Asia's Largest States, argues that 'in a marriage market where women are scarce and thus able to "marry up", certain characteristics of young surplus males are easily predicted' (Hudson and Den Boer). The pair argue that unmarried men are likely to come from the lowest socio-economic class, be un- or underemployed and live a fairly nomadic live with few ties to the communities in which they are working. The duo contends that a gender imbalance, caused by a shortage of marriageable women, results in higher rates of crime, including murder and rape, committed by young unmarried men who lack stable social bonds.

Violent crime in India rose nearly 19 per cent from 2007 to 2011, while the kidnapping of women (the majority of which is for forced marriage) increased 74 per cent in that time (Ministry of Finance, 2011).

The same report showed that of all the people arrested for rape, almost 60 per cent were men aged between 18 to 30 years (Ministry of Finance, 2011).

If the study's conclusions are correct, India's shocking problem with violence against women—which frequently makes the front page of newspapers across the country asking: why is this happening?—may only get worse. Given that Delhi has already been labelled the rape capital of the world, it's difficult to envision how much worse the situation could get.

'Where men will not be able to get married, it will lead to violence. It's hard to prove but there's reason to worry that violence against women will increase in one form or another,' Sital Kalantry, a professor at Cornell Law School, tells me.

'One wonders how connected the male surplus is to the violence that is happening in India now. Policy-makers are ignoring it. I would encourage the government to focus on the consequences of sex selection and take it more seriously than enacting laws and looking the other way.'

As men embark on a mission to secure a wife, and if women are able to 'marry up'—that is, beyond their caste and across state borders—how will these women be treated? Will they be subjected to more violence compared with the 33 per cent of married women who have already faced violence at the hands of their spouses? (International Institute for Population Sciences, 2017)

In a patriarchal society, where men hold much of the structural power, researchers suggest that the power imbalance, combined with the competition for the scarce number of women, indicates that men will be more likely to use violence to control women 'in order to limit their ability to form relationships or interact with other men who are in copious supply in the community' (Bose, Trent and South, 2014, p. 4).

Looking beyond the impact surplus men will have on women but on society as a whole, Hudson and Den Boer (2002) argue that India's surplus male population threatens domestic stability and international security. They suggest that a move to authoritarianism is far more likely and so is increasing sectarian and ethnic violence.

'In a way, the very type of government to which a nation can aspire may be tied to the status of women in society,' they write (2002). 'When that status is very low, the possibilities for a full and meaningful democracy and for a peaceful foreign policy are distinctly less.'

✳

Where are the men in all this? What is their role in perpetuating son preference and sex selection?

Countless studies have been dedicated to understanding why women opt for sex selection so much so that one would believe they are solely responsible for it. As a result, myriad policies and schemes aimed at women have been designed with the expectation they would stop women from seeking sex-selective abortions and using other sex-selective methods.

In stark contrast there have been few studies that have examined men's attitudes towards son preference. Moreover, research on men's roles in sex selection simply does not exist.

In a male-dominated society, where women have little autonomy and decision-making power within families, this is nothing less than striking. It is incomprehensible that extensive research has not been done to examine the extent to which men perpetuate son preference and sex selection.

Men not only play a critical role in shaping attitudes towards girls but are often the perpetrators—forcing women to undergo sex-selective abortion or to take sex selection drugs.

'Women are only considered breeding stock and men's honour. Sex selection is just part of the continuum of gender discrimination. The idea has to move out. In a patriarchal society, who can challenge an idea better than anyone else? Men,' Abhijit Das, co-chair of the Men Engage Alliance, a global network of organisations working on gender justice, and director of the Centre for Health and Social Justice (CHSJ) in New Delhi, says.

'Men together can create new social norms.'

Recognising that the sex ratio will not improve unless men are part of the fight, the CHSJ has trained 10,000 male 'gender champions' across several Indian states.[2]

The recruits undergo a six-month programme which involves group meetings, online training and theatre shows to educate men and create a sense of public outrage about their discriminatory behaviour. The idea, Das tells me, is that each gender champion will become a role model in his village and go on to create a group of his own.

The programme doesn't discuss methods of sex selection. It instead examines how men's actions are fuelling the declining sex ratio and looks at ways in which men can create new social norms.

'We talk about why the sex ratio is declining within the domain of gender discrimination without having a conversation about abortion. We think that the moment you focus on the womb, you are getting into women's reproductive rights,' Das says.

It's too soon to evaluate whether the programme is successful. But it is at least kick-starting a much-needed conversation.

[2] Part of this story has been published previously in Sophie Cousins, 'Don't commit the mistake I made': the men fighting India's female foeticide, *The Guardian*, 30 October 2018. Available at: https://www.theguardian.com/global-development/2018/aug/30/men-fighting-female-foeticide-india

Including men in the discourse on sex selection is not about publicly outing those who have propagated it. It's about getting men to reflect on their own behaviour. It's also about encouraging men who loathe gender discrimination to stand up and speak out against it. It's about realising that the issue of son preference and sex selection is not a women's issue; that it's a societal issue which is not going to be addressed by implementing laws and schemes that only target women.

※

For years, Dr Sutapa Neogi, a maternal and child health specialist at the Public Health Foundation of India, has been on the forefront of research into the impact sex selection drugs (SSDs) have on women. After being deemed a 'waste of time' by the male-dominated medical community for years, she has gone on to prove a clear link between consuming SSDs, stillbirths and birth defects. She's now on a mission to eradicate the practice.

On a sweltering afternoon in July 2018 I visit New Delhi Railway Station to witness Dr Neogi's latest project in real time. The station is jam-packed with thousands of people sprawled out on newspapers waiting for their trains. Everything is on offer at the station from books to bananas to rice cookers—and even television.

Ten times a day a film produced by Dr Neogi and her team pops up on television screens at railway stations across parts of north India where sex selection drug use is rife.

The short film begins at a hospital with a doctor telling a woman's mother-in-law and husband that she's very sorry, your wife has had a stillbirth.

It then flashes back to the family's living room and shows family members forcing the woman to take SSDs.

The purpose of the film is not just to educate some of the 23 million passengers on India's railway network every day, but to highlight the undue pressure women come under to produce a son.

'Apart from educating people about the drugs, we also have to highlight that women come under a lot of pressure from their husbands to take the drugs. Women face domestic violence if they don't deliver a son,' Dr Neogi tells me.

Dr Neogi is not so naïve that she expects a film to change people's mindsets, but in the absence of anyone else being as committed as she is to curbing the practice, she simply wants people to be aware.

'Taking sex selection drugs is unethical and people should be made aware of the dangers otherwise all of my research is pointless. I can't change people's mindsets but it's important that men know about this more than women because they're the decision-makers,' she says.

✳

Back at Meena's parents' house, after she has shown off her son Manish and put him down for a nap, I pull out my phone to show her the film that Dr Neogi has made. Network coverage is terrible in Behlba village so we wait about 15 minutes until the video, which is on YouTube, loads. That gives Meena's family and a few neighbours who have stopped in for chai ample time to crowd around to glare at the illuminated screen.

It's only a short film but everyone watches intently. Once it's over I ask Meena what she thinks about it.

'It's a good thing to have this issue in a form of a movie so people can actually be aware,' she says.

'But even if you tell people sex selection drugs are not good, people will still take them. People won't listen. No one will listen to me when I tell people these drugs won't give them a boy child. How can I convince them?'

Meena desperately wants no other woman to lose a baby like she did.

But the man of the house, Meena's father, has the final word.

'Getting people to stop sex selection is like asking a smoker like me to stop. You can tell me all about the health consequences but I'm not going to.'

References

Bose, S., Trent, K., and South, J.S. (2014) The effect of a male surplus on intimate partner violence in India. *Economic and Political Weekly*, 48 (*35*). Available at: https://www.ncbi.nlm.nih.gov/pmc/articles/PMC3914764/pdf/nihms 539069.pdf

Gargan, E. (1991) Ultrasound skews India's birth ratio. *New York Times*, 13 June. Available at: https://www.nytimes.com/1991/12/13/world/ultrasound-skews-india-s-birth-ratio.html

Guilmoto, C. (2012) Skewed sex ratios at birth and future marriage squeeze in China and India, 2005–2100. *Demography*, 49 (*1*): 77–100.

Hudson, V. and Den Boer, A. (2002) A surplus of men, a deficit of peace: Security and sex ratios in Asia's largest states, *International Security*, 4 (*26*), pp. 5–38. Available at: https://www.mitpressjournals.org/doi/10.1162/01622880 2753696753

International Institute for Population Sciences (2017) *National Family Health Survey-4 (2015–16)*. Ministry of Health and Family Welfare, Government of India. Available at: http://rchiips.org/nfhs

Manchanda, S., Saikia, B., Gupta, N. et al. (2011) Sex ratio at birth in India, its relation to birth order, sex of previous children and use of indigenous medicine. *PLoS One*, 6(*6*). DOI: 10.1371/journal.pone.0020097

Ministry of Finance (2018) Chapter 07- Gender and son meta-preference: Is development itself an antidote? *Economic Survey 2017–2018*, pp. 102–118. Available at: http://mofapp.nic.in:8080/economicsurvey/pdf/102-118_ Chapter_07_ENGLISH_Vol_01_2017-18.pdf

Ministry of Home Affairs (2011) National Crime Records Bureau: Prison Statistics India 2011. Available at: http://ncrb.gov.in/statpublications/psi/Prison2011/ Full/PSI-2011.pdf

Ministry of Statistics and Programme Implementation (2017) Youth in India, Government of India. Available at: http://mospi.nic.in/sites/default/files/ publication_reports/Youth_in_India-2017.pdf

Ministry of Women and Child Development (2015) Beti Bachao, Beti Padhao, Government of India. Available at: http://www.wcd.nic.in/bbbp-schemes.

Neogi, S., Negandhi, P., Chopra, S et al. (2015) Risk factors for stillbirth: Findings from a population-based case-control study, Haryana, India. *Paediatric and Perinatal Epidemiology*, 30(*1*): 56–66.

Neogi, S., Zodpey, S., Negandhi, P. et al. (2017) Use of sex selection techniques for social reasons: A menace. *Indian Pediatrics*, 54(*2*): 99–101.

Office of the Registrar General and Census Commissioner (2011) *Census of India: Our Census, Our Future*. Ministry of Home Affairs, Government of India. Available at: http://censusindia.gov.in/

Pande, R. and Malhotra, A. (2006) *Son Preference and Daughter Neglect in India*. International Center for Research on Women.

Planning Commission (2011) Report of the Steering Committee on women's agency and child rights for the twelfth five year plan, Government of India. Available at: http://planningcommission.gov.in/aboutus/committee/strgrp12/str_womagency_childrights.pdf

Portner, C. (2015) Sex-selective abortions, fertility, and birth spacing. Policy Research working paper, World Bank.

Sharma, N. (2010) Boy oh boy. *Hindustan Times*, 18 August. Available at: https://www.hindustantimes.com/entertainment/boy-oh-boy/story-eUeRMn9Ue8amoYv0iiNs5L.html

United Nations Office on Drugs and Crime (2013) Current status of victim service providers and criminal justice actors in India on anti human trafficking. Available at: https://www.unodc.org/documents/southasia/reports/Human_Trafficking-10-05-13.pdf

World Bank (2018) Fertility rate, total births per woman. Available at: https://data.worldbank.org/indicator/sp.dyn.tfrt.in

CHAPTER 2

Boys vs Girls
Child Mortality Inequity

The poorer you are, the closer you will live to Deonar landfill, Mumbai's largest open dumping ground. The dump, which receives hundreds of tonnes of waste every day, is so mammoth it can be seen from space. It's so putrid that it can be smelt miles away. And it's so toxic that people die from simply inhaling the fumes it emits. The normal lifespan of a landfill is 40 years; Deonar has been running since 1927, making it Asia's oldest landfill.

If you've just migrated to India's largest city, also known as the City of Dreams, from the states of Uttar Pradesh, Bihar or Karnataka, and you're a Muslim or a Dalit, it's likely you'll end up across the road from the landfill at Shivaji Nagar slum. The slum began as a resettlement colony where poor Muslim and Dalit communities from slum communities across Mumbai were taken and dumped like trash in the early 1980s. Since then it has mushroomed to accommodate more than 600,000 people, housing migrants and their families who come here in desperate search of work.

Mumbai is one of the world's most densely populated cities. Space is so limited at Shivaji Nagar, situated in the north-east of the sprawling city, that mounds of trash have to be flattened to make space for the never-ending demand for shelter. Despite Mumbai being the richest municipality in South Asia, it's not unusual to live in a slum. In fact, about 60 per cent of its 18 million inhabitants live in slums. The long-running joke is that the city—which derives its global fame from being the head-quarters of Bollywood—should perhaps be renamed 'Slumbai'. But the term slum is used loosely here; not everyone lives in the brightly coloured shanty-towns that have been sold to the West in movies, like the favelas of Brazil. Many homes that have been notified as slums by the government are actually built with bricks and cement and also have functional infrastructure like a regular water supply.

But the Shivaji Nagar slum is something else. Decades of government neglect has kept it in a perpetual state of precariousness.

It's a place where every day is a fight for survival—and even more so if you're a girl.

✳

It's the height of the monsoon season in July 2018 and I'm walking through Shivaji Nagar, stomping over piles of rubbish strewn everywhere. Sewerage runs through the slum's maze of narrow alleyways. The alleyways are so narrow that you're either going in one direction or the other—two people can simply not squeeze past one another.

The sewerage is so deep and thick, and the monsoon rain so frequent, that residents have had to build long wooden planks to put above the knee-deep chocolate-coloured water just to reach their one room homes. I pass one young boy who is bent over at the corner of one of the slum's main thoroughfares drinking sewerage water through a plastic straw. Safe drinking water is a luxury here.

There's a designated meat area in the slum—an area where families are preparing thousands of lunches for daily labourers who are working nearby in a range of jobs from construction to garment factories. Goats, cows and chickens surround the open kitchen where women are cooking fragrant curry in deep stainless steel pots. A group of men stand next to a pile of red onions almost as tall as the roof waiting for the food to be ready so they can deliver it on their bicycles.

Three of Nassrah Khatoon's daughters are outside the shop where she works, scrubbing their clothes and school bags with rags. Nassrah, who is wearing a deep purple headscarf, puts down her knife, and comes outside holding her one-and-a-half-year-old daughter in one arm. She has five daughters in total—the eldest is seven years old. Another child is on its way and due in five months' time.

All the girls have shaved heads because 25-year-old Nassrah simply doesn't have time to do their hair.

Six years ago Nassrah and her children migrated to Mumbai from Bihar, one of India's poorest states which borders the Himalayan nation of Nepal, because of a lack of job opportunities. Her husband had already moved to Shivaji Nagar many years ago.

The family of seven—soon to be eight—live in one room. Between Nassrah cooking for daily labourers and her husband delivering the food everyday, the pair make ₹6000 (US$86) per month. To make a few extra rupees her husband buys onions from outside Mumbai and sells them at a small mark-up inside the slum.

The family pay ₹1500 (US$22) per month for their home. They have a fan and one light bulb which costs a few dollars a month. They try not to rely on the fan to keep their place cool but Mumbai is incessantly humid.

They don't have a direct water supply so every day Nassrah waits for the water truck to arrive. When it does, it's a fight who in the community can get it and who can afford it. Nassrah's family buys one bucket of water every day at a cost of ₹50 (US$0.70). It's not enough to bathe every day but they make do.

Since Nassrah married nine years ago, at the age of 16, she's had children non-stop. As she likes to say, it's been 'bam bam', her fist pumping the air.

She didn't want to have this many children. But the problem is that she hasn't had a boy. So she's had to keep reproducing.

'It's necessary to have a boy. That's why I'm pregnant again,' she says.

'It's the mentality of the community that every family needs a boy so that's why I want a boy.'

Nassrah sits on the floor of a nearby community health centre not far from where she works. Her youngest daughter sprawls out across her swollen belly while the four others plays with one another. All the girls have swollen bellies like their mother.

The two youngest girls have severe acute malnutrition (SAM)—the most extreme form of under-nutrition—characterised by very low weight for their height and severe muscle wasting. Their bloated bellies are caused by a protein deficiency which causes an osmotic imbalance in the gut.

Her three other daughters have been categorised by local healthcare workers as having moderate acute malnutrition (MAM). In other words, they are malnourished but not to the grave degree to which the younger ones are.

Nassrah says her younger daughters are more malnourished than the older ones because she hasn't had time to take care of them. The more children she's had, the less time and money she's had to feed them sufficiently. She also didn't breastfeed the youngest.

'I had much more time to look after the older kids—to focus on them and feed them. But the more children I have, the less time I have. There's so many to look after plus cooking and cleaning that I don't have time to look after the kids,' she says.

For the last six months the children have been taking a form of Ready-to-Use Therapeutic Food (RUTF) that is used to treat malnutrition. It's a thick paste which is calorie dense, protein rich and fortified with essential micro-nutrients required for growth and weight gain. It includes ingredients such as peanut paste, milk powder, soybean oil and emulsifier. It's helping but the children aren't in the clear yet.

'I just feed them whatever food there is,' Nassrah says.

Meanwhile, Nassrah just eats the leftovers.

She points to her eldest daughter whose legs are bowed inwards because of rickets—a result of an extreme and prolonged vitamin D deficiency which causes the weakening of bones in children.

'She could barely walk because she was so weak,' Nassrah says.

*

While son preference in Indian society manifests itself in harsh and obvious ways such as sex-selective abortion, it can also manifest in subtler forms.

For the first time the Indian government's 2017–18 annual economic survey revealed there are 21 million 'unwanted' girls in India, a phenomenon known as meta-preference (Ministry of Finance, 2018, p.105).

Meta-preference involves parents adopting fertility 'stopping rules'—having children until the desired number of sons are born. Nassrah's case in point: once she has a son she will stop having children.

This meta-preference inevitably leads to the notion of 'unwanted' girls—girls whose parents wanted a boy, but instead had a girl. Often, like in Nassrah's case, women reproduce repeatedly over a short period of time in their desire to have sons. Many end up with six or seven children just in order to get a son.

While a son meta-preference doesn't lead to sex-selective abortion or female foeticide, it nevertheless can be detrimental to female children and their health.

More broadly, it begs the question: what happens to girls who are born and who survive?

*

India houses about half of the world's undernourished children.

The 2015–16 National Family Health Survey—a nationwide survey—shows that 38 per cent of children under five are stunted (short for their age); 21 per cent are wasted (thin for their height);

and 36 per cent are underweight (thin for their age) (International Institute for Population Sciences, 2017).

While the survey doesn't break down statistics by gender, one doesn't have to look far to see the inherent son preference and daughter discrimination playing out.

A leading hypothesis is that in a society with a deeply entrenched son preference, this partiality, which begins before birth, extends into childhood, with families giving boys more food than girls (Jawaregowda and Angadi, 2015, p. 507). And this discrimination begins at breastfeeding.

The benefits of breastfeeding cannot be overestimated. Breast milk doesn't only contain all the vitamins and nutrients infants need for their first six months of life, but it's packed with disease-fighting substances that protect babies from illness. In a setting like India where water-and food-borne illnesses are rife, exclusive breastfeeding is even more critical.

The recommended infant and young child feeding practices as per the World Health Organisation include exclusive breastfeeding for the first six months of life, continued until the age of two (World Health Organisation, n.d.). Solid and semi-solid foods that contain a variety of micronutrients should be introduced at six months and should be increased as the child ages.

The latest National Family Health survey found that 55 per cent of children under the age of six months are exclusively breastfed (International Institute for Population Sciences, 2017).

Research shows that on average Indian girls experience about one-half month shorter breastfeeding duration than boys (Fledderjohann et al., 2014). Researchers from the University of Oxford and the London School of Hygiene and Tropical Medicine found that second-born girls were the most likely to receive the least breast milk (Fledderjohann et al., 2014). Girls, they discovered, were also less likely to have received breast milk and fresh milk as a source of protein in the last 24 hours compared with boys.

Receiving less breast milk may not sound like a major issue. But shorter periods of breastfeeding are not only associated with a higher risk of stunting, but it also increases the chance of an infant dying from respiratory and diarrhoeal diseases (Jayachandran and Kuziemko, 2009, p. 23).

In fact, the researchers found that the longer infants are breastfed, the greater the survival benefits, with each month of breastfeeding reducing the risk of dying by 24 per cent (Fledderjohann et al., 2014).

But not all girls get to reap the vast benefits of breast milk.

So why would girls be breastfed less than boys?

Numerous factors could affect a mother's tendency to breastfeed which could be completely unrelated to her child's gender, including her health status, the availability and affordability of breast milk substitutes, and her participation in the workforce (Jayachandran and Kuziemko, 2009, p. 1). But one critical factor that cannot be ignored is that breastfeeding is a natural contraceptive. What does that mean in the context of having a daughter or two or three?

Researchers from the National Bureau of Economic Research in the United States found that after the birth of a daughter, mothers were more likely to want to continue having children and thus limit breastfeeding in order to conceive again (Jayachandran and Kuziemko, 2009, p. 1). This finding correlates with the meta-preference phenomenon—having children until a son is born, or the desired number of sons is born.

That means that so long as a preference for a son exists, some boys will be breastfed longer than girls. Shorter durations of breastfeeding will inevitably fall on the girl child because, as the government's economic survey 2017–18 revealed, Indian families tend to 'stop' having children after a son is born or when they have their desired number of sons (Ministry of Finance, 2018, p.1).

Jayachandran and Kuziemko conclude that boys are, overall, breastfed for longer periods of time which is 'a result consistent with mothers valuing boys' health more than girls' health or simply wanting to be more loving towards sons' (2009, p. 21).

Health and nutritional discrimination has far-reaching consequences for girls. It could begin to explain why India is the only country in the world where young girls have worse under-five mortality than boys and why declines in infant mortality have been far greater in boys than girls.

✳

Asarfi's new cement home was meant to represent hope—hope of a better future. From the outside, it certainly stands in stark contrast to her chocolate-coloured mud-brick home with a thatched roof that sits next to it. Her new home is made of cement and red-bricks and has a hardened roof to protect her family from the monsoon rains. But inside is a sad story of government neglect.

On the front wall of the home is an oversized red sign in Hindi which reads, 'Prime Minister['s] Rural Housing Scheme'.

But only part of the money to build the home as part of Prime Minister Narendra Modi's promise to build 30 million homes for the poor by 2022 has been received. The family, like many others in neighbouring villages, hasn't received new instalments.

Inside the home is a small cook-stove in the corner with a few onions and a handful of rotis next to it. They haven't received any money to furnish the home, let alone lay down all the cement. The remainder of the home is bare except for three thin pink shawls that the family lie on top of at night.

It's June 2018, and I'm in Mehra village in the central Indian state of Madhya Pradesh.

Madhya Pradesh is in the heart of India where the majority of its 74-million-strong population is dependent on agriculture. It's also a state with a large Scheduled Castes (SCs) and Scheduled Tribes (STs) population—people who are the most socio-economically disadvantaged in India. Under British rule, they were known as the

Depressed Classes; in Hindu society, despite laws that aim to create equality, they are still relegated to the lowest rung of society.

Mehra village is about a three-hour drive from the state's most northern city, Gwalior, in the Shivpuri district. It could be a faster trip if it weren't for the herds of cattle that park themselves conveniently on the highway. Herders whack the cows and buffalo with long bamboo sticks in an attempt to get them moving. But the heat is debilitating and the animals are tired.

Madhya Pradesh is by no means considered a tourist destination. But Gwalior Fort, situated on top of a hill above the dusty city, is breathtaking, particularly at dusk when the glowing red sun sets behinds its walls. The fort's inscriptions represent the city's ancient past which date back to at least the tenth century.

Mehra village is a series of thatched huts, mud-brick homes and a few unfinished cement and red-brick houses. The surrounding land is sparse; tall trees make way for the reddened earth and provide some reprieve from the oppressive heat.

Asarfi and her husband, Ramraj, don't exactly know their age, but guess they're between 28 and 30 years old. Both their families have lived in Mehra village for generations.

The couple are migrant daily labourers. They work half the year ploughing the fields of Madhya Pradesh earning ₹150 (US$2.20) per day. In November, when their work at home dries up, they migrate to the northern state of Uttar Pradesh or the western state of Rajasthan to plough wheat, soya beans and potatoes. In Uttar Pradesh and Rajasthan they are at the mercy of the owners of the field. They don't get paid in cash; instead their income is received in bucket loads of wheat. They work the fields during the day and in the evenings sleep in a makeshift tarpaulin tent, their heads nestled in between the crops, the smell of dirt-covered potatoes lingering in the brisk air.

It's work that they're used to—their parents did it and so did their grandparents.

The couple have two children: a son who is 13, and a daughter who is seven. Their son is tall and is wearing a plaid light blue shirt, dark denim jeans and a caramel coloured belt. Their daughter is wearing a tattered pink and gold-coloured dress with an oversized bow on the front. Her hair is ear-length and her belly bloated.

Six months earlier, on 20 January, the couple's 16-month-old daughter died. Her name was Poonam.

'Poonam was malnourished for seven or eight months. She died at home,' Asarfi says.

'I tried to feed her but she vomited everything. She didn't eat roti or anything.'

Asarfi doesn't have many memories of Poonam, but she does vividly remember buying her daughter a pomegranate just days before she died. It was expensive but she'd been told the fruit was packed with vitamins. She had cracked open the fruit and fed her daughter a few bright purple pearls of sweetness before she vomited them back up.

Poonam wasn't the family's first child to die.

In June 2017, Sanam died. Sanam was another of the couple's daughters. She was three years old.

Within just six months two daughters had died.

And at some point in 2015—Asarfi can't remember exactly when— Shri Devi, another daughter, died. She too was three years old.

'We have had three deaths in the family. They all died of malnutrition,' Asarfi tells me.

'Because my baby died again I don't want to have any more children.'

Sitting under a tree outside their home, Asarfi's husband, Ramraj, explains the repeated tragedies in the simplest terms.

'Why the three girls died in this house is that the boy is the eldest. After him, there was less work, less money and more mouths to feed. We had so many mouths to feed and because the boy was the eldest, he got good care,' he says.

The family doesn't have anything but their memory to remember their three daughters by. They have no photos—not even the passport-sized ones that many families carry in their wallets—no old clothing, no favourite toys.

The move into the family's new home at the end of 2017 was meant to be a new start—an opportunity to move on from the deaths of their two daughters. It was meant to resemble hope and prosperity.

✳

Ajay Yadav has been working on the issue of malnutrition in Shivpuri district since 1990. He's a tall, slim bespectacled man who is soft-spoken and profoundly gentle. His presence is immediately calming and it's easy to understand how he has developed such strong bonds with the communities he works with.

Yadav says discrimination against girls here extends far beyond nutrition and is often so nuanced that it requires close scrutiny.

'In this community they say they don't prefer boys over girls but the preference is seen. There's a difference in the type of clothes parents provide to sons compared with daughters,' he says.

'Daughters are also the first ones to go out and work. Families prefer their sons to go to school every day but don't let their daughters go because they're usually kept at home for work.'

Asarfi breastfed her son for two years and her daughter for one year.

Their daughter, Delva, doesn't go to school—she's kept at home to do household chores. When she's 10, her father, Ramraj tells me, she'll be sent to a city to work.

'For our son,' Ramraj says, 'it's his wish. Whenever he wants to work, at 15, or later, then he can. Whatever is his wish. If he doesn't want to work, then we won't pressure him.'

✳

As per the latest National Family Health Survey (2015–16), 38 per cent of Indian children are stunted—too short for their age (International Institute for Population Sciences, 2017).

The astronomically high figure means that one in every three stunted children around the world lives in India (Jayachandran and Pande, 2017, p. 2600).

Child stunting is a key marker of child malnutrition and is driven by poor nutrition and repeated infection. On average, people who are shorter as children are less healthy, have lower cognitive ability, poor educational performance, low adult wages, and lost productivity (de Onis and Branca, 2016). The World Health Organisation labels child stunting as one of the most significant impediments to human development (2014, p. 1).

Two development economists—Professor Seema Jayachandran from Northwestern University in Illinois and Professor Rohini Pande from Harvard Kennedy School in Massachusetts—recently examined the records of almost 170,000 children in India and 25 African countries (2017, p. 2603). They were on a quest to understand why India has a perplexingly high rate of stunting. It inevitably led them to investigate the role that gendered parental preferences play.

Their analysis of child height-for-age data found that firstborn boys in India are taller than their African counterparts (Jayachandran and Pande, 2017, p. 2603). More importantly, they found that Indian parents' unequal allocation of resources across children affects their height and that height disadvantage among children starts with the second child and increases sharply with birth order (2017, p. 2600).

Data on height for girls and boys at different birth orders supports their theory. For example, a son who is the second child is taller in India than Africa if his older sibling is a girl. If a girl has an older brother, then it's likely she is going to fare far worse in terms of health and nutrition. They also found that relative to sub-Saharan Africa, girls in India receive fewer postnatal resources if their family does not yet have a son (Jayachandran and Pande, 2017, p. 2306).

'We propose that eldest son preference in India—encompassing both a desire to have at least one son and for the son to be healthy— influences parents' fertility decisions and how they allocate resources across children, leading to the steep birth order gradient in height,' the economists wrote in their study published in the *American Economic Review* (Jayachandran and Pande, 2017, p. 2602).

While on paper greater financial resources could enable families to provide children with enough food and adequate healthcare to achieve their height potential, the economists were sceptical that inequality across birth order would diminish because it has continued despite widespread economic improvements.

'Parents' son preference and unequal investment in children do not seem to be diminishing,' they wrote (2017, p. 2626).

✳

India is the only country in the world where girls have a greater risk of dying under the age of five than boys (Fledderjohann et al., 2014). And India and China are the only two countries in the world where female infant mortality (dying under the age of one) is higher than male infant mortality.

Because of biological and genetic reasons, boys up to the age of five are more likely to die than girls. They are weaker and more susceptible to diseases and premature death.

But India appears to be an exception to the rule.

An analysis of sex differentials in child mortality across 150 countries by the United Nations Department of Economic and Social Affairs (UNDESA) found that an Indian girl aged between one and five years is 75 per cent more likely to die than an Indian boy of the same age (United Nations Department of Economic and Social Affairs, 2011).

The analysis, which tracked infant and child mortality rates from the 1970s to 2000s, found that in the 2000s, there were 56 under-five male child deaths for every 100 female child deaths (United Nations Department of Economic and Social Affairs, 2011).

It showed that the disparity between female and male child deaths had only worsened over time. For example, in India in the 1970s, 75 boys under-five died for every 100 girls; in the 1980s, the ratio was

69 boys for 100 girls (United Nations Department of Economic and Social Affairs, 2011).

In contrast, for the rest of the developing world (83 countries), in the 1970s, 111 boys under-five died for every 100 girls (United Nations Department of Economic and Social Affairs, 2011). By the 2000s, that ratio had increased to 119 boys for every 100 girls.

The analysis indicates that not only do females have a distinct advantage in survival up until the age of five, but that such an advantage has continued to increase as infant and child mortality has declined across the developing world. But in India, girls have not benefited from such survival advantages.

The report attributes the significantly higher mortality of girls to 'differential treatment in regard to preventive and curative healthcare as well as feeding and nutrition' (United Nations Department of Economic and Social Affairs, 2011). It calls on the plight of girls in India to remain in the 'global spotlight'.

But the disparities in child mortality cannot just be explained by feeding and nutrition differences.

According to the latest data from the United Nations Children's Fund, almost 1.1 million children under five die in India every year (UNICEF, 2011). Excluding deaths among neonatal babies—those who die within the first month of life—the major causes of death include pneumonia and other respiratory infections, diarrhoea, malnutrition, malaria and other non-communicable and communicable diseases (Bassani et al., 2010).

Hundreds of thousands of these deaths could be prevented if children had access to nutritious food, clean water, sanitation, vaccinations and prompt medical treatment, including simple antibiotic treatment.

But girls face rampant gender discrimination when it comes to preventing illness and when it comes to treating it.

✳

With the exception of the development of antibiotics, no other public health innovation has had the same impact as vaccines.

Vaccines have drastically reduced disease, disability and deaths across the world from numerous communicable diseases including diphtheria, measles, mumps, whooping cough, Haemophilus influenza type b, pneumonia, polio, rotavirus diarrhoea, rubella, and tetanus.

According to India's third National Family Health Survey in 2005–2006, 44 per cent of children aged 12–23 months had received the basic vaccinations which include one dose of BCG vaccine, which protects against tuberculosis; three doses of DPT vaccine, which protects against diphtheria, pertussis (whooping cough) and tetanus; three doses of the polio vaccine; and one dose of the measles vaccine (International Institute for Population Sciences, 2007). By the latest National Family Health Survey in 2015–16, that percentage had increased to 62 per cent (International Institute for Population Sciences, 2017).

The survey didn't take into account the other vaccinations that are now also part of the country's Universal Immunisation Programme (UIP). They include the pentavalent vaccine, introduced in 2015, which protects against the three diseases in the DPT vaccine in addition to hepatitis B and Haemophilus influenza type B (a bacterium which causes meningitis and severe pneumonia in children); rotavirus, which was introduced in 2016; and pneumococcal, introduced in 2017.

Again, however, girls face widespread discrimination when it comes to receiving vaccinations.

An analysis of three rounds of the National Family Health Survey undertaken between 1992 and 2006 found that girls are less likely to receive vaccinations at any given age compared with boys (Corsi et al., 2009). The researchers found that birth order and family composition is an important predictor of vaccination coverage. Girls who are born third into a family of two girls face 'extreme' vaccination disadvantage compared with boys who are born third into families with two older girls (Corsi et al., 2009). For example, just 36 per cent of third born girls with two older sisters are given basic vaccinations (Corsi et al., 2009).

The study found the three states with the lowest girl-to-boy ratios of vaccination coverage are the northern states of Punjab, Haryana and Bihar—states with India's most skewed sex ratios and thus the strongest preference for sons (Corsi et al., 2009).

'Gender inequity in access to health programmes is responsible for a considerable number of avoidable deaths. India's states could save even more lives by addressing deep-seated social and cultural issues responsible for gender discrimination at the household level, where girls are seen as a burden and boys as a resource,' the researchers concluded (Corsi et al., 2009).

One doesn't have to look far to look at the impact vaccine discrimination has on girls. In fact, Emily Oster, a professor of economics at Brown University in Rhode Island, estimates that between 20 and 30 per cent of excess child female mortality can be attributed to vaccination bias (2009). Because most vaccinations do not take place until an infant is between six and 12 months (often later than the recommended age of dose), Oster highlights that this contributes to the acute excess female child mortality between the age of one to five—a time where the impact of missing out on life-saving vaccinations would emerge (2009).

'There has been significant focus in India on changing preferences— for example, encouraging people to put greater value on women, promoting female schooling, and so on,' she wrote (2009). 'These are clearly useful goals. However, in the shorter run... investments in vaccination for girls would have a direct effect on excess female mortality... [A] focus on universal vaccination would have the largest effect on mortality.'

While the latest National Family Health Survey shows an increase in basic vaccination levels, one can only expect that discrimination against girls will continue unabated. The recent inclusion of the pentavalent vaccine in the programme, along with rotavirus and pneumococcal vaccine, is a unique opportunity to prevent tens of thousands of child deaths every year from pneumonia, diarrhoea and

Haemophilus infuenza type B. But whether girls will benefit from the inclusion of these vaccines in the UIP to anywhere near the same degree as boys remains to be seen.

✳

Rajnandini is 15 months old but she doesn't look older than just a few months. Her head is as round as a cherry tomato and disproportionately larger than her skeletal body which sinks into an oversized beetroot- and gold-coloured dress. She's wearing three beaded necklaces around her neck, one navy bracelet and another string on her ankle. It's good luck, her grandmother tells me.

Rajnandini is so thin that her belly is not bloated like the traditional images of malnourished children; instead her bones protrude out of her skin. Her arms and legs are as wide as a banana and her eyes are sunken into the back of her head. Rajnandini's mother holds her in one arm, but she's so fragile that she's almost swallowed up beneath her mother's purple sari.

I'm still in Madhya Pradesh at a village called Pohari. It's about a 20 minute drive from Mehra village where Asarfi and her family live.

There's no road into Pohari. To reach the village you either need an off-road vehicle or to walk a few kilometres from the main road.

It's the height of the monsoon season and the sky is dark and threatening. Grey clouds hang low as sun beams occasionally try to squeeze through to shine light onto the rich earth.

The fields surrounding the village are lush and the small brown water inlets are almost overflowing.

About 100 people live here in mud-brick homes with thatched rooves. Bricks are carefully positioned on top of the rooves to protect families from the heavy downpours they experience.

Children run around the village barefoot as young girls congregate on charpoys to pick lice out of one another's hair. Young men pass the time by listening to their favourite Hindi songs on a shared mobile.

Like Mehra village, Pohari also has a few new cement homes that have been built under Narendra Modi's Rural Housing Scheme. Villagers had thought that finally someone was paying attention to the plight of their village. But new homes have been forgotten, left half constructed after the remaining funds to finish building were never received.

For the last few months Rajnandini has had recurrent diarrhoea, fever and vomiting. Yellow snot has been dripping into her mouth for weeks so much so that Ramglassy, her mother, no longer bothers to wipe it off her philtrum before she swallows it.

The family, which also includes their four-year-old son, recently returned from work in the western state of Rajasthan where they were ploughing fields. For the remainder of the year Ramglassy and her husband will cut grass in the neighbouring fields for work.

Sitting outside the family's mud-brick home, Ramglassy gets up to lay her daughter down inside. Their rounded clay hut is bare except for a few old yellow rice bags that lay strewn across the floor and a cook-stove in the corner. Rajnandini lies on top of a rice bag, using her hands as a pillow, and stares into the distance trying to catch her breath in between her crying. Flies swarm her delicate body but she's too tired to flick them away.

Ramglassy steps outside and sits down under a nearby tree. She knows her daughter will eventually fall asleep. Meanwhile, her four-year-old son, who is wearing jeans and a shirt, is laughing while playing on a mobile phone with his cousins.

Ramglassy is fully cognisant that her daughter is facing death if she doesn't get medical treatment quickly. One can learn a lot about a village by asking who has recently died. And this village has seen too many deaths.

It was only last week that a family in the mud-brick home directly across from Ramglassy's family lost a baby due to malnutrition and tuberculosis.

She says she hasn't taken Rajnandini to the hospital because it's four kilometres away. That means she'll have to pay for transport.

It will also require time away from work, meaning a loss of income for the day.

'Look at her,' malnutrition activist Ajay Yadav—who is travelling with me today—pleads with Ramglassy. 'She's very serious. She's needs medical care or she will die.'

Other villagers wobble their heads in agreement.

After about half an hour of pleading with Ramglassy, she finally gives in.

'Ok I will bathe her tomorrow and bring her to the hospital.'

✳

What happens when a child gets sick in India? Do parents seek timely medical treatment—which is technically free at public healthcare facilities—equally for both sons and daughters? Are parents willing to spend the same amount of money on medical care, such as medicines and transports costs, for both girls and boys?

Research shows that qualified healthcare providers are consulted more often and sooner for boys, and that parents are willing to travel longer distances for sons (Pandey et al., 2002). In contrast, less money is spent on healthcare for girls. Moreover, girls, particularly infants, are more likely to die at home without getting any medical attention at the last critical time of their lives in both urban and rural areas across India (Asfaw, Klasen and Lamanna, 2007, p. 7).

The Indian census as early as 1901 noticed the less notorious but more far-reaching benign neglect that girls are subjected to. 'There is no doubt that, as a rule, she [a girl] receives less attention than would be bestowed upon a son. She is less warmly clad, ... She is probably not so well fed as a boy would be, and when ill, her parents are not likely to make the same strenuous efforts to ensure her recovery' (Mudur, 2016).

History continues to repeat itself.

One could conclude that widespread poverty across India, particularly in the north, prohibits families from seeking timely medical care for their children and that it was just a coincidence that Asarfi's three daughters died at home in her arms. But research shows that even among the poor, the probability of boys being hospitalised when they're sick is far higher than girls (Saikia, Moradhvaj and Bora, 2016). For sons, parents are more willing to look for alternative financing such as borrowing money from family, friends or moneylenders (Saikia, Moradhvaj and Bora, 2016). In other words, gender discrimination in delays in seeking healthcare, along with healthcare expenditure, thrives across all socio-economic groups for both serious and minor illnesses from pneumonia to a bout of diarrhoea.

It is difficult to comprehend why a mother would not want to save her child's life. Looking at Rajnandini's helpless, frail body lying on an old rice bag, I wondered why her mother needed so much encouragement—and to a certain extent pressure—to take her dying daughter to a hospital that was only a few kilometres away. Was it really down to the fact that she already had a son who was strong and healthy and Rajnandini was simply a burden on the family? Perhaps. Was it that taking her daughter to the hospital would take up too much time—time that she couldn't afford to miss earning money on the fields? Perhaps. Was it that taking her daughter to the hospital required agency and involvement in decision-making? Perhaps. Maybe it's a combination of all three factors and a whole lot more.

But more than that, Ramglassy has been brought up in a society where women's lives are not as valued as men's; a society where women lack agency and empowerment, where everything they do is for the males in their families. Perhaps she was subconsciously projecting her own experiences onto her daughter and putting her daughter's health last—just like her own.

✳

The next afternoon I visit the malnutrition ward four kilometres from Ramglassy's home. She promised that we'd meet again there.

The three-level clinical white coloured hospital is unusually quiet and uncharacteristically orderly. A few people trickle in through the doors; some are pushed in on wheelchairs, others are carried by loved ones. I'm led upstairs to the malnutrition ward where about 15 women lie on metal gurneys, cradling their babies in their arms.

I scan the room, hopeful that I'll meet Ramglassy's eyes. But she's nowhere to be seen. I walk back and forth down the narrow hospital ward, my sandals scraping the white tiled floors, turning my head slowly from left to right making sure not to miss a single woman. I can't find her. I get a sinking feeling in my stomach, a realisation that Ramglassy was never going to come.

Like Ramglassy's daughter, the infants at the ward are severely malnourished. All but one is female. Their bodies are so weak from dehydration that their cheeks appear hollow like a pumpkin on Halloween and they are so exhausted that just a few manage a soft cry.

A whiteboard hangs above each gurney which records every child's weight. Some weigh no more than a few kilograms.

At the ward both mother and child are fed runny dal, rice, roti, porridge and a selection of fruits including papaya, pomegranate and bananas for two weeks. Many babies subsist on Ready-to-Use Therapeutic Food (RUTF), an energy-dense micronutrient paste used to treat severe acute malnutrition, which Nassrah's children in Mumbai are also fed. For many of the mothers here it's the first time they've ever cut open a papaya let alone popped open a pomegranate to suck on the pearls of sweetness.

The goal of the malnutrition ward is to bring the infants back from the brink of death and increase their weight. But it's when the mother and her child are discharged that the real challenge begins.

Sitting on the last bed in the corner of the long narrow room is 30-year-old Lata. She's been at the hospital for the last 12 days with her 10-month-old daughter Rasali. She has two other daughters and a son who is the eldest at five years. Lata travelled 50 kilometres to the hospital after a local healthcare worker insisted she come or her daughter would face the prospect of death. When she arrived disconcerted, her daughter was vomiting violently.

Rasali has never tasted breast milk and often Lata gives her water from a dirty well. Coming here for two weeks is a big commitment— Lata has forfeited two weeks of daily labouring work to care for her daughter.

In the last 12 days, Rasali has put on 800 grams—a phenomenal amount of weight given she only weighed about four kilograms when she arrived. The pair are leaving in two days' time for their arduous journey home and Lata hopes she can put into practice what she's learnt here. But vegetables and fruits are expensive, as she knows, and she's not lactating.

'I'm anaemic. Just before I gave birth to Rasali I found out I was anaemic. I will try to do things differently when I leave the hospital. It will be hard but I'll try,' she says.

I ask all the other women in the room if they too are anaemic and one by one they all wobble their heads.

*

Anaemia is a condition in which the number of red blood cells or their oxygen-carrying capacity is insufficient to meet physiological needs. Under-nutrition, specifically iron deficiency, is the most common cause of anaemia around the world, though other deficiencies including vitamin B12 and vitamin A, along with parasitic infections and chronic inflammation, can also cause it.

Anaemia can lead to fatigue and loss of energy, shortness of breath, difficulty concentrating, dizziness and insomnia. More concerning though is the inter-generational impact it has on women and their children, particularly girls.

As of 2016, more than 50 per cent of pregnant women across the country are anaemic and one in four is undernourished (International Institute for Population Sciences, 2017). According to the latest National Family Health Survey, 59 per cent of children under five are anaemic (International Institute for Population Sciences, 2017).

Women's poor nutrition, both before and during pregnancy, contributes significantly to impaired foetal development and contributes to low birth weights, which in turn leads to high rates of stunting (Vir, 2016).

Widespread nutrition deprivation among women perpetuates an inter-generational cycle of nutrition deprivation in children, particularly girls. Undernourished girls grow up to become undernourished women who give birth to a whole new generation of undernourished children. Moreover, severe anaemia is a major contributor to postpartum haemorrhage, the leading cause of maternal deaths in India.

Under-nutrition and anaemia is not simply about a lack of food. It's so much more than that. It's a symptom of social inequality. It's about gender inequality, stigma and discrimination, a lack of education and decision-making, and a lack of investment in nutrition of self, children and family.

For example, a woman who has been married off as a child at the age of 10, who has lacked access to education and nutritious food as a child, who has conceived as a teenager, who has little agency in her family, who always eats last, is likely to give birth to a low weight child. If she's a girl child, she will be likely to face the same dire consequences of being a female and so the cycle continues.

'It's an intergenerational cycle,' Ajay Yadav says as we sit under the tree outside Asarfi's home in Mehra village.

'You see Asarfi was married at 10. She has given birth to six children so far, three of which have died. You can see her condition. Will she be able to give birth to a healthy child? No.'

Asarfi tells me that when she last gave birth—to her baby Poonam who died at the age of 16-months—she was told she was anaemic. She doesn't really know what that means except that she's meant to eat more. That hasn't happened, though.

'After cooking, I always eat last. I eat four or five rotis a day. Sometimes I have roti with chutney but that's it,' she says.

'I'm anaemic and because my baby died again I don't want to have any more children but I don't know what family planning is.'

* * *

Back in the maze that is Shivaji Nagar slum in north-east Mumbai, heavy rain is battering the bruised tin rooves. People huddle under shop fronts while others run to grab red buckets to place inside their homes underneath leakages. The rain hasn't deterred a group of children who are lined up outside a local organisation waiting for their name to be called. One by one each child is weighed, and their legs and arms measured before they open their tiffin, ready for a few scoops of salty peanuts.

Almost 50 per cent of children in the slum are stunted and one in five is wasted, local healthcare workers tell me. Malnutrition hits girls much harder than boys, they add.

'No priority is given to girls' nutrition here—far more preference is given to boys,' Sunita Choure, a local healthcare worker, says.

As soon as the peanuts are scooped into their tiffins, the boys sit down and start munching. Girls on the other hand put the lid on their tiffins and hold them preciously like they're carrying gold and navigate the narrow alleyways back to their homes. I ask healthcare workers why the girls don't sit down to eat their peanuts. Girls, I'm told, must bring the peanuts home to share with the family; boys, on the other hand, are allowed to eat them straight away.

It's a nuanced difference but one that is emblematic of the stark gender inequality and discrimination girls face and how the intergenerational cycle of malnutrition continues.

'A girl is stunted not because there is a lack of knowledge or because parents are not sensitive, but because of the larger socio-political-cultural issues that families find themselves in generation after generation,' Arun Kumar from Apnalaya, an organisation that works on delivering healthcare in the slums of Mumbai, says.

✳

Nassrah Khatoon rubs her belly and then her feet. She knows she's meant to eat more nutritious food when she's pregnant, especially since she's anaemic. But with five malnourished girls and full-time strenuous work cooking all day, it's a constant struggle.

She just desperately hopes her next child will be a son so she can stop reproducing.

'My wish is that at least two of my children be educated. I won't be able to afford all their education so if at least two of my kids are educated I will be really happy,' she says.

Before we finish talking, her mobile phone rings. She doesn't pick up. It rings again and again, until she eventually picks up.

'Hello,' she says.

'Come home. I'm hungry,' her husband replies.

References

Asfaw, A., Klasen, S. and Lamanna, F. (2007) Intra-household gender disparities in children's medical care before death in India. IZA Discussion Paper No. 2586. Available at: https://pdfs.semanticscholar.org/5d3a/6ce4a54bd6e c18875f8d785f2ca5820cff6b.pdf

Bassani, D. G. and Jha, P. (2010) Causes of neonatal and child mortality in India: nationally representative mortality survey. *The Lancet* 376 (*9755*): 1853–1860. Available at: https://www.thelancet.com/journals/lancet/article/PIIS0140-6736(10)61461-4/fulltext

Corsi, D., Bassani, D. G., Kumar, R., Awasthi, Shally, et al. (2009) Gender inequity and age-appropriate immunization coverage in India from 1992 to 2006. *BMC International Health & Human Rights* 9 (*Suppl 1*):S3. Available at: https://doi.org/10.1186/1472-698X-9-S1-S3

de Onis, M. and Branca, F. (2016) Childhood stunting: A global perspective. *Maternal & Child Nutrition* 12:12–26. DOI: 10.1111/mcn.12231

Fledderjohann J., Agarwal S., Vellakkal S., et al. (2014) Do girls have a nutritional disadvantage compared with boys? Statistical models of breastfeeding and food consumption inequalities among Indian siblings. *PLoS ONE* 9(9): e107172. Available at: https://journals.plos.org/plosone/article?id=10.1371/journal.pone.0107172

International Institute for Population Sciences (2007), *National Family Health Survey-3 2005–06 (Volume- I)*, Ministry of Health and Family Welfare, Government of India. Available at: https://dhsprogram.com/pubs/pdf/frind3/frind3-vol1andvol2.pdf

International Institute for Population Sciences (2017) *National Family Health Survey-4 (2015–16)*. Ministry of Health and Family Welfare, Government of India. Available at: http://rchiips.org/nfhs

Jawaregowda, S. K. and Angadi, M. M. (2015) Gender differences in nutritional status among under five children in rural areas of Bijapur district, Karnataka, India. *International Journal of Community Medicine and Public Health* 2(4): 506–509. Available at: https://www.ijcmph.com/index.php/ijcmph/article/viewFile/1007/875

Jayachandran, S. and Kuziemko, I. (2009) Why do mothers breastfeed girls less than boys? Evidence and implications for child health in India, National Bureau Of Economic Research. Available at: https://www.nber.org/papers/w15041.pdf

Jayachandran, S. and Pande, R (2017) Why Are Indian Children So Short? The Role of Birth Order and Son Preference. *American Economic Review* 107(9): 2600–2629. Available at: https://www.aeaweb.org/articles?id=10.1257/aer.20151282

Ministry of Finance (2018) Gender and son meta-preference: Is development itself an antidote? *Economic Survey 2017–2018*, pp. 102–118. Available at: http://mofapp.nic.in:8080/economicsurvey/pdf/102-118_Chapter_07_ENGLISH_Vol_01_2017-18.pdf

Mudur, G. S. (2016) Even educated spend less on women health. *The Telegraph*, 7 July 2016. Available at: https://www.telegraphindia.com/india/even-educated-spend-less-on-women-health/cid/1516840

Oster, E. (2009) Proximate sources of population sex imbalance in India. *Demography* 46(2): 325–339. DOI: https://doi.org/10.1353/dem.0.0055

Pandey, A., Sengupta, P. G., Mondal, S. K., et al. (2002) Gender differences in healthcare-seeking during common illnesses in a rural community of West Bengal, India. *Journal of Health, Population & Nutrition*. Available at: https://www.ncbi.nlm.nih.gov/pubmed/12659410

Saikia, N., Moradhvaj. and J.K., Bora. (2016) Gender difference in health-care expenditure: Evidence from India human development survey. *PLoS ONE* 11(7): e0158332. Available at: https://journals.plos.org/plosone/article?id=10.1371/journal.pone.0158332

United Nations. Department of Economic and Social Affairs- Population Division (2011) *Sex Differentials in Childhood Mortality*, United Nations Publication. Available at: http://www.un.org/en/development/desa/population/publications/pdf/mortality/SexDifferentialsChildhoodMortality.pdf

United Nations International Children's Emergency Fund (2018) *Under-five Mortality*, United Nations. Available at: https://data.unicef.org/topic/child-survival/under-five-mortality

Vir, S. C. (2016) Improving women's nutrition imperative for rapid reduction of childhood stunting in South Asia: Coupling of nutrition specific interventions with nutrition sensitive measures essential. *Maternal & Child Nutrition* 12: 72–90. Available at: https://www.ncbi.nlm.nih.gov/pmc/articles/PMC5084747/

World Health Organisation, *Breastfeeding*, United Nations. Available at: https://www.who.int/nutrition/topics/exclusive_breastfeeding/en/

World Health Organisation (2012) *WHA Global Nutrition Targets 2025: Stunting Policy Brief,* United Nations. Available at: https://www.who.int/nutrition/topics/globaltargets_stunting_policybrief.pdf

CHAPTER 3

From Birth to Death
The Maternal Death Road

The naked baby boy stands on his two feet, wobbling from side to side. His arms extend awkwardly outwards towards a photograph his grandmother is clasping tightly in her wrinkled, sun-drenched hands. He tries to grab it, but falls over into a pile of cow dung. He gets back up and tries again, wiping the slimy poo off his petite legs. He reaches for the passport-sized photograph again, unaware that his arms are not long enough. Sensing his impending distress, his grandmother Jamuna Sharma, picks him up and rocks him gently. For a brief moment the two forget about the beloved person in the photograph and embrace tightly. But then it hits them, like a mammoth wave crashing against a struggling swimmer and tears flood their faces, tears so heavy that the little boy has to gasp for air.

The photograph, which is small enough to hold between two fingers, is of Seema Devi.

Seema was the little boy's mother and Jamuna's beloved daughter-in-law. She died giving birth on 31 March 2018. She was just 24 years old. The photograph is the only meaningful object the family has to remember Seema. For two-year-old Upendra, it's the only visual connection he has to his mother.

I'm in Sahabganj, a small town in the northern state of Uttar Pradesh in Chandauli district, about a two hours drive south-east of Varanasi. Sahabganj is what is known as a 'block' in India—a cluster of several neighbouring villages—and is surrounded by sprawling fields of rice and wheat.

We're sitting in the family's brown-brick cow shed on plastic chairs on top of a mound of hay. Next to us is the family's prized spotted white and brown cow. Behind the cow shed is a wide brick courtyard which branches off into three separate rooms where the extended family sleep and cook. The cow shed is the coolest spot, one that offers some respite from the oppressive heat.

Uttar Pradesh is India's most populous state with more than 200 million people. It's home to the majestic Taj Mahal, the red-brick walls of Agra Fort and the spiritual capital of India, Varanasi, which attracts millions of Hindu pilgrims every year to bathe in the scared water of the Ganges River and perform funeral rites.

It's also home to the second highest rate of maternal mortality in India (National Institution for Transforming India, 2018). Early on March 31, Seema Devi began having painful contractions. It was time. She'd been advised by a village female healthcare worker known as an auxiliary nurse midwife (ANM) to give birth at a private hospital about 30 kilometres away. The ANM, who lived just a few houses down from the family, was a trusted member of the community. She worked at the local health sub-centre, a small village-level health institution, and received a government salary. She'd advised Seema throughout her pregnancy. Seema not only felt comfortable with her, but depended on her wisdom.

The family knew that giving birth at a private facility would be costly, but they also knew that government-run facilities, particularly in rural areas, lacked quality care. Often there would be no doctors available; other times people would wait hours on end to be seen, only to be told the medical tests they needed were not available or that they needed to go elsewhere. Plus, the private hospital was closer to the family home.

The family put into action their plan: Seema's father-in-law, Ganga, would rent out the family's land for ₹30,000 (US$420) over the next year. It would be more than enough to pay the private hospital fees and put some aside. The decision to rent out their land wasn't taken lightly—it would severely hamper the family's earnings from crops for the next year. But under the guidance of the ANM—a government healthcare worker who receives 18 months' training—they were encouraged to do so. Doubts about quality aside, her advice came despite services at public healthcare facilities being free and programmes run by the government which give women living under the poverty line money when they give birth at a public facility.

Seema's husband, Virendra, was unable to help. He was far away working in Mumbai where he'd been for the last five years because of a lack of job opportunities in Sahabganj. He didn't know that six months ago, when he last visited his wife and rubbed her tummy, that it would be the last time.

There was no ambulance available to take Seema the 30 kilometres to the hospital. It refused to travel down the graveled, pot-holed road to their home. The family ordered a taxi and waited. When they arrived at the hospital they paid ₹4000 (US$56) for admission.

Seema was howling in pain. While she'd given birth before, her family knew this pain was something different. Something wasn't right.

She was screaming for the nurses to help, to do something, anything, and for a doctor to come and see her.

For hours her screams went unanswered.

'The nursing staff were forcing her to have a normal delivery. They kept saying, "It is a normal case and let the normal delivery happen." There was no doctor. The nurses told me that if an operation was needed, then a doctor will come and operate on her,' Jamuna, Seema's mother-in-law, says.

It wasn't until 24 hours later, when it was clear that no doctor was coming to help Seema, that a nurse told the family that Seema's condition was serious and that they could not help. The healthcare workers not only failed to recognise Seema's complications, but they wasted critical time before bothering to tell her family.

Seema's blood pressure had dropped drastically and she was bleeding. She was referred to a hospital two hours away in Varanasi. By the time she got there, Seema was dead and so was her baby. Her baby died in her womb. It was an intrapartum foetal death.

Before breaking the devastating news to the family, the hospital had the audacity to charge them ₹12,000 (US$168) for 'hospital fees' including medicines and medical tests they'd never heard of.

'Seema was healthy. She was strong enough to handle the delivery but because there were no doctors she died,' Jamuna tells me, wiping the heavy tears off her cheeks.

'If a caesarean section would have happened then she could have been saved.'

✳

'Women are not dying because of a disease we cannot treat. They are dying because societies have yet to make the decision that their lives are worth saving,' Mahmoud Fathalla, then-President of the International Federation of Gynaecology and Obstetrics, told a conference audience in Copenhagen in 1997 (United Nations Secretary-General, 2013).

While there have been significant improvements in maternal health since Fathalla made those comments, maternal deaths remain one of the greatest injustices of our time.

Maternal mortality is a reflection of women's status in society. After all, it is only women who can experience maternal mortality. And in India, an estimated 44,000 women die from preventable pregnancy-related causes every year. While the country has made huge progress in reducing its maternal mortality rate from 556 per 100,000 live births in 1990 to 130 per 100,000 live births in 2016, huge disparities between states, rural and urban areas, and the rich and poor remain (Singh, 2018).

The major causes of deaths are postpartum haemorrhage (severe bleeding after childbirth); infections; eclampsia (high blood pressure during pregnancy); unsafe abortion; and complications from delivery. The largest share of deaths occurs during delivery; the remainder take place earlier or in the postpartum period (Singh et al., 2009, p.3). From a medical standpoint, most deaths are preventable if women receive the care they are entitled to in an effective and timely manner.

But these deaths are not solely a result of biological and individual risk factors. They are a combination of structural and social determinants such as the low status of women, poverty and a lack of transport, among myriad others.

A fundamental problem with aggregating data into one figure—a nationwide maternal mortality rate (a figure which is widely disputed in itself)—is that it not only doesn't tell us who the women dying are, but it also doesn't tell us exactly how they died.

Moreover, their medical records, which just document the biological cause of death, only capture a small, fragmented part of their story. The 44,000 women who die during or after childbirth every year are just a number on a dusty government report, the root causes of their deaths go ignored and their stories remain unheard. Most of these deaths inevitably take place in the most impoverished rural and remote parts of the country which are out of sight of policy-makers.

'The tragic reality is that too often maternal deaths are not visible. They don't leave any trace behind, and their deaths are not accounted for,' a report titled India's Silent Tragedy says (United Nations Children's Fund, 2008). While death is the most extreme outcome, government figures also neglect the fact that for every woman who dies, an estimated 20 more suffer from infection, injury and disability connected to pregnancy or childbirth (United Nations Children's Fund, 2008).

✳

In a bid to improve infant, child and maternal mortality and morbidity the Indian government, under the National Health Mission (formerly the National Rural Health Mission), runs three core health-care programmes.

Launched in 2005, Janani Suraksha Yojana (JSY) is a programme that aims to reduce maternal and neo-natal mortality by promoting institutional delivery among poor pregnant women through conditional cash transfers.

The government believed that if women gave birth at an institution—as opposed to at home where unattended, unsafe births remained common—deaths would drastically decline.

After delivery in a government facility or one of the few accredited private health facilities, eligible women receive between ₹700 (US$9.80) and ₹1400 (US$19.60) depending which state they live in and whether they live in a rural or urban area. The programme is centred on the ten 'high-focus states' including Uttar Pradesh, Bihar, Uttarakhand, Jharkhand, Madhya Pradesh, Chhattisgarh, Assam, Rajasthan, Odisha and Jammu and Kashmir, where all women irrespective of socio-economic status are eligible for the cash benefit. It's these states which have the highest levels of maternal mortality and the lowest levels of institutional births.

In the non-high focus states women are eligible for the cash benefit for their first two births and if they have a government-issued below-the-poverty-line card or if they are from a Scheduled Caste or Tribe. The health facilities are meant to pay incentives into the mother's bank account at the time of discharge.

To reduce out-of-pocket expenses, antenatal and postnatal check-ups, vaccinations and transport services to and from healthcare centres are also technically free.

The programme is supported in the community by Accredited Social Health Activists (ASHAs) who form the backbone of India's healthcare system. Based in their own communities, ASHAs are local women between the ages of 25 and 45, who act as an interface between their community and the public healthcare system. The 800,000-strong workforce doesn't receive a salary, but instead relies on cash incentives for their work. An ASHA worker's tasks include encouraging women to have an institutional birth, promoting vaccination, encouraging and mobilising access to family planning, and educating the community on nutrition. They also accompany women during labour and conduct postpartum visits. Under JSY, ASHAs receive ₹600 (US$8.40) for referring a woman to a public health facility to give birth in a rural area and ₹200 (US$2.80) in an urban area.

Launched in 2011, the Janani Shishu Suraksha Karyakram (JSSK) supplements JSY by offering free services to all pregnant women and sick neonates and infants at government institutions. The scheme envisions healthcare to operate completely cashless by providing pregnant women with services including normal delivery and caesarean sections, along with medicines, diagnostics, transport and food for free at all public healthcare facilities across the country. Under the scheme, sick newborns and infants are entitled to free healthcare too.

The third programme, the Integrated Child Development Services (ICDS), was launched in 1975. The scheme targets children up to the age of six, in addition to pregnant and lactating mothers with complementary nutrition. The ICDS operates through a network of 1.3 million Anganwadi centres. The centres, which are located within a few kilometres of villages across the country, provide complementary nutrition, schedule immunisations, distribute vitamin A, iron and folic acid tablets, and treat minor ailments. The centres are run by an Anganwadi worker, a local woman who has undergone a three-month training in child development, immunisation, breastfeeding, treatment of minor illnesses and recognition of 'at-risk' children.

✳

The JSY is the largest conditional cash transfer system in the world, with more than 50 million beneficiaries as of 2015 (Sabde, 2016). On paper it appears to be doing what it set out to achieve: to increase institutional births. In 2005, 38.7 per cent of women gave birth at an institution (International Institute for Population Sciences, 2006). By 2015–16 that figure had increased to 78.9 per cent (International Institute for Population Sciences, 2017).

JSY was formulated under the assumption that institutional births—deliveries in health clinics and hospitals—were far safer than home deliveries because of the availability of trained healthcare professionals and emergency obstetric care. Recognising that poor women—who have the least access to skilled care—bear the brunt of maternal mortality, the primary purpose of the programme is to incentivise women for a free delivery, thereby overcoming financial barriers to seeking healthcare.

The programme, however, has been plagued by severe shortfalls. For one, it relies on trained healthcare workers to not only actually be available but to be able to recognise danger signs. It also relies on essential infrastructure in the most far-flung areas of the country and basic commodities like drugs being available, along with a strong referral service when needed. But what has emerged across large swaths of India is a programme that places little focus on safe delivery and quality care; a system that fails to approach maternal health from a human rights perspective.

Research shows that JSY doesn't translate into safer, and dignified births and thus a reduction in maternal mortality (Randive, Diwan and De Costa, 2013). While it's clear that the programme has increased institutional deliveries, experts argue that the conditional cash transfer scheme disproportionately attracts pregnant women without complications to health facilities (Randive, Diwan and De Costa, 2013). In other words, women who are most likely to die in childbirth are not entering the programme.

Research also shows there is a lack of skilled birth attendance, a failure to carry out emergency obstetric care in obvious cases of need and a weak referral system (Chaturvedi et al., 2014). While the programme is designed to alleviate the financial barriers women face in choosing where to give birth, red tape related to women actually receiving the cash incentive is threatening to also undermine the programme. Stories of women not receiving the incentive are bountiful.

One study found that while women who entered the JSY programme paid less compared with women who delivered at home, they did not have a free delivery as intended by the public healthcare system (Sidney et al., 2016). It found that only one in four eligible women who delivered at a public health facility received the cash incentive upon discharge (Sidney et al., 2016).

In a 2014 piece published in the *New England Journal of Medicine*, researchers found that JSY didn't give credence to quality of care which in the end deterred patients from seeking care in public health facilities (Scott, Phil and Jha, 2013, p. 4).

'A puzzling issue confronting many policymakers is why, when formal public healthcare delivery systems are available (and often free), patients pay out of pocket to seek care from private providers... Despite broad consensus that patient-centered care is important, patients' actual experience falls far short of the ideal. When people are not treated with basic dignity and respect by providers, they are likely to avoid future interactions with those providers. Thus, even if care is safe, effective, and widely available, it is of little use if patients choose not to use it' the researchers wrote (Scott, Phil and Jha, 2013, p. 4).

The frequent failure of the healthcare system to care for pregnant women raises the question: what is the point of offering women cash to deliver in poor quality facilities without first ensuring quality of care and guaranteeing women they and their families will not be paying out of pocket? It is no wonder so many women are turning to the private sector. But it too is failing women, just like Seema.

*

In 2015, six hours after arriving in pain at a government hospital in Godda, a district in the eastern Indian state of Jharkhand, a doctor finally consulted Surujmuni Marandi, who was in labour.

Twenty-four hours later a nurse delivered her baby. She was charged ₹400 (US$5.60) for the delivery.

As Surujmuni was recovering from her difficult and prolonged labour, she spent all her money on hospital fees including medicines, toilet visits and tea. It wasn't long before she was left without a single rupee in her pocket.

When she next had to use the bathroom she had no option but to defecate in the open.

It was not supposed to be like this.

Surujmuni was supposed to receive ₹1400 (US$19.60) for giving birth in a government facility as part of the JSY programme. She was also meant to give birth, receive medicines, food, and transport to and from the government hospital for free as part of the JSSK programme.

She didn't receive anything for free.

But instead of resigning to the systematic failings of India's healthcare system, a video is produced about Surujmuni's struggles.

It's August 2016 and I'm travelling eight hours from Jharkhand's dusty capital Ranchi to Godda district to meet one of the women at the forefront of the fight against the state's unacceptably high rate of maternal mortality.

Ranchi is a city of just over one million people and is the gateway to the Betla National Park. The city, with its never-ending advertisements of English courses and call centre jobs, is emblematic of the youth's aspirations: to work or study in the places they've seen in Bollywood films. In sharp contrast to the aspiring English speakers who live in Ranchi are the millions more who live in the impoverished rural and remote areas. The Scheduled Tribe population of Jharkhand is just over seven million, constituting almost one-fourth of the state's population (Government of Jharkhand, n.d., p.1).

The 32 tribes of Jharkhand have been sorely neglected for decades. It is no surprise that the state has one of the country's highest maternal mortality ratios (National Institution for Transforming India, 2018).

The winding trip to Godda is filled with varied landscapes from rich green jungles, to desolate sandy brown land and vast, expansive coal mines. The state is rich in minerals—it has abundant reserves of iron ore, manganese ore, coal, limestone, lead and nickel. Children, men and women push rusted bicycles along curving roads piled with coal weighing hundreds of kilograms. Across the state an estimated 45,000 cycle wallahs transport 7.5 tonnes of coal each day. They push loads for up to 150 kilometres in the blistering sun or torrential rain, often barefoot or in oversized torn sandals, to a village or town where the coal will be traded at one rupee a kilo.

The sun is fire-red in the early evening in Godda district as it sets slowly behind the lush green rice paddies and sweeping palm trees. To the beat of drums a group of women swing their hips and dance towards a mud-brick shelter where dozens of locals have gathered on the floor for a video screening. There's only one light bulb in the shelter where people have gathered so many use the torches on their simple phones to find space on the floor to sit.

The film they have gathered to watch is about Surujmuni Marandi's experience of giving birth at their local hospital.

The eight-minute video, shot by local woman Mary Nisha, provides a heart-rending insight into the failings of the healthcare system in India for poor pregnant women—failings that are so common that women around the room wobble their heads as if they've witnessed it or been through it all before.

The most disturbing part of the film is when one of Surujmuni's relatives helps her hobble outside to defecate right next to the toilet. Humiliated and wincing in pain, she bends down to relieve herself. The film is so confronting and so horrifying that it's difficult to watch. Women's faces around the room show a mix of utter disgust and sheer disbelief.

At the end of the film, Mary Nisha, the filmmaker, tells the audience: 'I made this film because I consider any woman's problems as my own. My community and I want the poor [not to] be charged any medical services at the district hospital.'

When the film is finished women openly discuss their own birthing experiences. One after another they raise their hands and then their bodies, to tell their stories.

What emerges are dozens of similar stories of women repeatedly being denied hospital admission and being asked to pay for services. Numerous stories of women dying from postpartum haemorrhage and anaemia, two of the major causes of maternal deaths across the world, also emerge, told by widowers.

The women here in Godda believe they don't receive adequate healthcare services not only because they're women but because they are from what is considered the lowest rung in Hindu hierarchal society. One doesn't have to look far to see how this discrimination is impacting the women here. For example, in 2010, women from the Santhal tribe in Godda had a maternal mortality rate of 325, locals tell me. This stands in stark contrast to the state average of 212 and the country average of 130 in 2016 (Singh, 2018).

Mary Nisha is a feisty woman who made the video about Surujmuni Marandi's birthing experience. She's a former lands-rights activist turned maternal health activist. She was inspired to become the latter after she delivered her first two children at a government hospital. She was harassed by staff, pressured to give birth on a dirty aluminium birthing bed and forced to pay for her medical expenses. She was surprised she survived, let alone her children.

'Whenever I went to the government hospital, there were no facilities. It wasn't clean and people don't take care of you there,' she tells me in her open kitchen adjoined to her mud-brick home in her village in Godda.

'Whatever I'm doing for the health of women, I recognise myself in these situations. My heart is troubled and that is the only reason I do this work.'

The following day I travel four hours to the north-eastern town of Madhupur in the Deoghar district of Jharkhand to hear and watch more stories about the neglect of women's health.

In 2013, Aamna Bibi went into labour. She lived in a village not far from Madhupur, where the district hospital is located. Her family called for an ambulance to come and get her. It never arrived. Hours later when she arrived at the hospital after her family eventually found enough money for a taxi, she saw two empty ambulances sitting idly by the doors.

Aamna was screaming in pain. The pain was so bad that she was bent over like an elderly woman with severe osteoporosis. Two relatives had to help her walk through the hospital's corridors. Three hours later still no doctor had arrived. There was no one to help.

When the pain became unbearable and she could no longer hold out hope that a skilled healthcare worker would bother to turn up, the family felt they had no option but to borrow money and hire a taxi to take her to a private facility.

She didn't make it in time. Her baby was a stillbirth on the way.

A young local man, Mukesh Rajak, made a video about Aamna's horrific experience.

'Nobody else should face what I have gone through,' she tells viewers.

The most harrowing part of the five-minute video is watching the dead baby wrapped in white be buried.

Not long after Aamna's tragedy, another local woman, Kalima Bibi took her pregnant daughter who was in labour to the same hospital. When they arrived, the gates were shut and tightly bolted. An hour later a nurse opened the gates to those who urgently required medical attention. There was no doctor in sight.

A nurse delivered Kalima's grandchild but shortly afterwards her daughter began to bleed profusely. The nurses said they couldn't help and that Kalima must take her to a hospital in Deoghar, more than an hour's drive away. There was no ambulance so the family borrowed money for a taxi. Kalima's daughter and grandchild died on the way.

These harrowing stories, which have only come to light because people have broken their silence to fight against the structures that inflict this violence, again highlight why it's only the poor who rely on public health facilities.

✳

It has been widely recognised that health outcomes are not just a result of biological and individual risk factors but also of other factors like wealth, education and gender.

As such, it's critical to look at maternal deaths not only through the lens of a lack of healthcare services, but also through the other structural and social determinants of health.

A discussion paper by the United Nations Development Programme uses a framework to analyse the determinants of maternal health which is split into intermediary determinants of health, and structural determinants of health (2011). Intermediary determinants of health include individual attributes of women like age, parity and knowledge of services; family characteristics including economic status, access to resources and marital relationship; community context which includes social position (class, caste, ethnicity), social capital and distance to facilities; and health services which include availability of services, skilled staff and fees for services (UNDP, 2011). The structural determinants of health include governance and policies, including laws and reproductive health and rights; and cultural and social values which include women's status, gender norms, agency and health beliefs (UNDP, 2011).

This is by no means an exhaustive list of all the factors that influence maternal health outcomes but it nevertheless illustrates that the vast disparities between women globally cannot be explained by biological factors alone.

In 2012, the Dead Women Talking Initiative was launched by the Coalition for Maternal-Neonatal Health and Safe Abortion. The Coalition is a group of organisations and individuals in India focused on drawing attention to the unacceptably high levels of maternal mortality and the subsequent lack of transparency in the documentation of deaths. The Initiative seeks to expose and highlight the social determinants of maternal health, particularly women's low status in society and bring to the fore the voices of women who have died. Through telling women's painful stories, the Initiative presents compelling evidence why India's maternal health policy should move away from the paradigm of institutional deliveries to that of safe deliveries.

The Coalition analysed 124 maternal deaths across 10 states between January 2012 and December 2013 to illustrate that women's lack of decision-making, a lesser value placed on their lives and gender-based health disparities fuels maternal deaths (Subha, Sri and Khanna, 2014, p. 17).

While the individual stories of women dying from giving life are harrowing enough in itself, when looked at as a whole the analysis presents a broader story of a vicious cycle of early marriage, young pregnancy, pressure to reproduce because of son preference, gender inequality, and malnutrition. It also highlights the way in which the healthcare system propagates these issues by routinely failing to provide adequate antenatal and postnatal care.

'The health system could have responded in multiple ways in mitigating some of the problems these women were facing. Instead, we find that it miserably failed in doing so,' the report says (Sri and Khanna, 2014, p. 19).

Of the 124 deaths the group analysed, 78 women were under 25, and 26 of those women were under 20 years old (Sri and Khanna, 2014, p. 15). It is well known that women who face pregnancy at a young age face a higher risk of morbidity and mortality. Yet despite this widespread knowledge, the narratives reveal that numerous women didn't receive any antenatal care whatsoever during their pregnancy and among those who did, care was of extremely poor quality. The WHO recommends a minimum of four antenatal care visits for women with low-risk pregnancies (2016, p. 12). While antenatal care by itself cannot prevent maternal deaths, it plays a critical role in identifying, diagnosing and treating high-risk health problems before childbirth, including anaemia.

The latest National Family Health Survey shows that only 21 per cent of women receive full antenatal care which includes at least four antenatal visits, at least one tetanus toxoid injection and iron and folic acid tablets or syrup taken for 100 days (International Institute for Population Sciences, 2017). Under the National Health Mission (which was initially the National Rural Health Mission), a government initiative to address the health needs of under-served rural areas, a Village Health and Nutrition Day (VHND) is meant to be held once a month at Anganwadi centres, located in every village. The VHNDs are a critical opportunity to provide antenatal check-ups for pregnant women, in addition to identifying and referring women with severe anaemia (Intra Health, 2012). But such days don't appear to have come to fruition.

Anaemia was the cause of 22 deaths and contributed to at least four more out of the 124 deaths in the analysis (Sri and Khanna, 2014, p. 41). Anaemia also exacerbates the effects of postpartum haemorrhage, the leading cause of maternal deaths in India. Given India's extremely high rate of anaemia among pregnant women—50.4 per cent—it is astonishing that the detection and treatment of anaemia continues to be ignored (International Institute for Population Sciences, 2017). As the Initiative writes, 'It is... well-known that women with moderate to severe anaemia need special care during labour and delivery so they do not bleed excessively and that these women are at risk of cardiac failure in the hours immediately after delivery. However, the poor quality of care in health facilities seemed to mean that women did not in fact receive such care. We find that no concerted efforts have been made to address anaemia' (Sri and Khanna, 2014, p. 43).

Women, particularly poor, marginalised women, continue to be failed by the health system, to die of preventable causes, and be neglected by society. So who is to blame for the 44,000 maternal deaths in India every year? And can those responsible be held accountable? The Coalition has an idea.

'By making policies that actively exclude vulnerable women, by not building in mechanisms to make sure programmes are implemented, by allowing providers in the public sector to refuse care, by allowing them to violate all ethical norms of care, by allowing referral systems to treat women like footballs, by not demonstrating enough will to save women's lives. The state has to be held accountable for the deaths of these women,' the Initiative says (Sri and Khanna, 2014, p. 53).

✳

The sweeping tea gardens in the north-eastern Indian state of Assam are brilliantly beautiful. The emerald green, lush plantations extend for as long as the eye can see with women appearing as dots on the horizon carrying the next generation of tea workers on their backs.

Assam produces 51 per cent of India's tea and is the largest tea-growing region in the world (Arya, 2013). But while the verdant tea gardens of Assam are renowned for their beauty, the living and working conditions are a far cry from the pretty visuals gracing tea boxes. Every box of Assam tea sold internationally by tea giants, such as Lipton and Tetley, is picked by tea garden workers who work long, arduous hours in the cruel heat for about US$3 a day. The British brought the Adivasi communities, also known as the tea tribes, from the neighbouring states of Bihar and Odisha more than a century ago. The tea tribe community is estimated to number about six million—20 per cent of Assam's population according to the latest census (Office of the Registrar General and Census Commissioner, 2019).

The tea gardens, for all their splendour, speak to global, national and local inequality; the long-lasting effects of colonialism; the impact of globalisation; and the consequences stigma and discrimination has on women. The Adivasi community continues to face intergenerational oppression, fuelled by unremitting exploitation by tea garden management and the subsequent neglect by the government.

This is most evident in Assam's maternal mortality rate, which is the highest across India and almost double the national average at 237 deaths per 100,000 (National Institution for Transforming India, 2018). Experts tell me that up to 77 per cent of maternal deaths every year in the state are in the tea gardens.

But the true burden of deaths is unknown because too often tea garden worker deaths are not recorded.

＊

On a rainy afternoon in August 2015, I'm at the maternity ward at Assam Medical College in Dibrugarh, also known as India's Tea City, in the eastern part of the state. The industrial city is surrounded by expansive tea estates and sits along the Brahmaputra River, a trans-boundary river which also flows through Bangladesh and China.

For weeks I'd been trying to speak with women working in the tea gardens but my efforts had been thwarted. I'd been allowed into one tea garden to speak with a woman but the manager insisted that he stand idly by and monitor our interview. This made the young, pregnant woman I wanted to speak with extremely uncomfortable and reluctant to talk about her situation.

The overcrowded maternity ward is an insult to the senses: the stench of blood, sweat and dirt lingers in the hallway. The walls are covered in grimy green mould, the bed sheets are filthy and the floors are covered with streaks of mud and blood. There are at least three women to a bed as relatives sit amid the grime on the hospital's floors.

Twenty-eight-year-old Dungdin is seven months pregnant with her first child. She's underweight; her eyes are sunken deep into the back of her head and her frail body is almost too thin to hold up her red sari.

Dungdin works in one of the region's 800 tea gardens. She was brought to the hospital with placental abruption which resulted in the placental lining separating from her uterus.

Her immediate concern though is not her or her baby's health. Instead she worries about the wages she'll miss while in hospital and hopes to be discharged soon.

'I was working until the minute I came here and I'll have to work the minute after I give birth,' she says. 'I have no option.'

On the bed opposite her lies another young tea garden worker, 20-year-old Anjali, who was 31 weeks pregnant when she arrived at the hospital a few days ago.

'I wasn't feeling my baby move … I just found out the baby died in my uterus, so it will have to be removed,' she says.

✳

Why are so many women dying in the tea gardens of Assam?

While there is a dearth of data related to maternal deaths in the tea gardens, anaemia and pre-eclampsia have emerged as the leading causes of death (Hazarika et al., 2017).

More than 95 per cent of adolescents in the tea tribes in Dibrugarh district are anaemic (Mahanta et al., 2015). Diets low in essential nutrients but high in salt, tobacco and alcohol consumption are common among tea workers. This can lead to pre-eclampsia which occurs when women develop high blood pressure during pregnancy. If it's left untreated it can result in seizures and in areas like rural Assam where women have little access to quality healthcare, these complications can be deadly. Severe anaemia can weaken uterine muscular strength and lower resistance to infectious diseases which contributes to postpartum haemorrhage (Kayle et al., 2008). It can also cause cardiac arrest and is a contributor to other maternal deaths caused by eclampsia and sepsis (Sharma and Shankar, 2010).

Pre-eclampsia and anaemia are a product of entrenched poverty, a lack of education, social mobility, and access to healthcare, under-nutrition, early marriage and multiple young pregnancies. Every tea garden is legally bound to have a hospital on-site, but they are often ill-equipped with drug and staff shortages.

'The tea gardens have hospitals but there are no doctors. If you increase education, then people will demand more, but it's in the management's best interests to not improve education levels,' Dr B. C. Bora, who worked as a doctor in the tea gardens for almost a decade, tells me.

To counter anaemia, there are three government initiatives targeting low-income pregnant women: the provision of iron and folic acid tablets, nutritional supplements/rations given at Anganwadi centres and blood transfusions as needed. But these interventions, while promising on paper, do not function as outlined in the guidelines.

For the lucky ones who can afford to hire a taxi to Assam Medical College, the largest hospital in the region, it can involve hours of travel on poor, pot-holed roads. And when they get there, they are not guaranteed quality care.

'We are promoting hospital deliveries but this hospital (Assam Medical College) is not efficient enough. I can't say we're providing good services. We're completely overburdened. The conditions are horrible and the smell is horrible,' Tulika Goswami Mahanta, associate professor of community medicine at the college, tells me shaking her head.

'These deaths are preventable. A lot more women die than we realise.'

One critical, life-saving intervention for women with anaemia is adequate access to blood. But for tea garden women access to blood during delivery is all but a distant dream. Research has found that many tea garden women were only given blood after they had provided replacement blood through a donor (Sachdev, 2018) If women do not have a blood donor, they end up paying exorbitant fees. 'This system has serious impacts on women's health, particularly [for] those who are unaware of the need for a donor, or [are] unable to pay for one. It not only causes delays, but it also narrows the options of treatment made available to women,' the research reads (Sachdev, 2018).

Simran Sachdev, justice programme officer at Nazdeek, a legal empowerment organisation based in New Delhi, tells me that the blood transfusion issue highlights the injustice tea garden workers face.

'Women in the tea gardens face so many barriers for a safe delivery. So many cannot afford a blood transfusion that they go home without it. The blood is rightfully theirs but hospitals let women go home and die. This issue encapsulates all the issues women in tea gardens face,' she says.

'Wage plays a big role in this issue. Any nutrition needs go to the bottom of the priority list.'

On my last day in Assam I visit Sandip Ghosh, secretary of the Assam branch of the Indian Tea Association (ABITA), which represents the industry. ABITA works with UNICEF to provide nutrition counselling and promote institutional deliveries through awareness programmes in the tea gardens, along with educating adolescent girls on issues including delaying marriage. I ask him why maternal deaths are so unacceptably high; why, despite the interventions he's laying out to me, they are not budging year after year.

'We can't change minds that are set. That is why we're targeting adolescents. But it makes business sense to have healthy workers,' he tells me.

Instead of drawing on the vicious cycle of stigma and discrimination, of oppression and poverty, and of social immobility and a lack of local health services, Ghosh shifts the blame to women. It is women and their narrow minds that are to blame for dying during childbirth.

*

India has made unprecedented strides in getting women to deliver in institutions, spurred on, one would assume by government programmes—JSY and JSSK—which are supposed to provide women with free deliveries and for those who qualify, conditional cash transfers.

According to the National Family Health Survey 2015–16, overall institutional births in India stand at 78.9 per cent (International Institute for Population Sciences, 2017). But just 52.1 per cent of these take place at government health institutions and the remainder take place in the private sector (International Institute for Population Sciences, 2017).

The reasons for this are multifaceted but almost universally tie back to the same issue: the failure of the healthcare system to care for women. Desperate to get some form of care in the face of an often unresponsive health system, some feel they have no option but to turn to the private sector. But such a decision propels countless families into debt.

For those who believe that the private sector provides exemplary medical care—that paying a high price secures quality care—may be in for a rude shock. The sector operates completely unregulated and with no regulation comes a lack of accountability.

The private sector is driven by money and thus arise critical questions of to what degree providers exploit the poor, those who are propelled into debt to pay for often unnecessary services from blood tests to CT scans.

As K. Sujatha Rao, a former union secretary of the Ministry of Health and Family Welfare argues, 'Society as a whole seems to have lost its soul in its blind pursuit of making money ... the health sector has been reduced to profiteering, be it in the area of medical education or providing services' (Rao, 2017, p. xx).

Back in Sahabganj in Uttar Pradesh and encouraged by their local ANM worker who was overseeing Seema Devi's pregnancy, her family-in-law mortgaged the land they live off to be able to afford private healthcare. But money could not buy Seema's safe delivery.

The family was sceptical about the provision of care in the public sector, but their decision to turn to the private sector was ultimately driven by the ANM worker who persuaded the family it was in their best interest.

But what unfolded was a disaster: staff failed to recognise classic obstetric emergency warning signs and failed to refer Seema to another facility in a timely manner. When she arrived dead at the second private facility, the hospital had the gall to charge the family an extraordinary ₹12,000 (US$173).

Why would an ANM worker—who is employed by the government and thus paid a government salary—encourage a woman to give birth in a private facility?

At first it made no sense. But it does now.

What has emerged is an elaborate private sector scam that involves everyone from taxi drivers, to government-employed healthcare workers, all the way up to head doctors.

Jashodhara Dasgupta, founder of SAHAYOG, an organisation that works on maternal health and rights, says that the flourishing private sector thrives on a lack of government services to exploit the poor. She explains that village level workers, ASHAs and ANMs, are paid more money than their government incentives or small salaries to send local women to private facilities.

'The entire story of the availability of services is critical here,' she says.

'Poor families are trying to ensure that childbirth is safe but the health system is failing to save women's lives.'

Given that ASHA and ANM workers' pay is so skeletal, Dasgupta asks a pertinent question: Why wouldn't they take money from the private sector?

The private sector, like the public sector, is failing women and will continue to do so until the whole system and those who participate in its operations are held accountable. Until women are able to access the care they need in a timely and efficient way, deaths will continue unabated. This is not only about addressing the fundamental shortfalls of the public and private healthcare sector but the deep-seated social determinants of health which, in India, mean that women's lives are not as valued as men's.

But instead of waiting for the healthcare system to be held accountable, some women are doing it for themselves.

✳

Back in Godda district in the eastern state of Jharkhand, Mary Nisha, the woman who had produced the horrifying film about Surujmuni Marandi's birthing experience at their local hospital, is packing her bag for the day's work ahead.

It's early morning and the blood orange sun is rising over the rice paddies as she makes some chai before leaving. In her bag are her reporting essentials: a notepad, pen and her small video camera.

Mary Nisha is part of Video Volunteers, a non-profit organisation that trains Indians from the lowest castes in the poorest parts of the country to tell their stories through video—stories that would otherwise go unheard.

The point of producing videos is not merely to give people a platform to be heard and to encourage people to take action, it's about the notion of community monitoring in the world's largest democracy.

One way to understand the importance of creating a movement around the 'right to voice' is through journalism scholar Michael Schudson's pivotal work. He argues that citizens are morally obliged to monitor powerful institutions from governments to corporations (Schudson, 2011, p. 309). It is in this sphere of monitorial democracy that women like Mary Nisha can produce reports, kick-start community discussions and ultimately advocate for change. At the end of her film about Surujmuni's horrific experience, Mary asks viewers to call the head doctor at the hospital and demand women be given the services they are entitled to. It may sound like an insignificant act but providing basic services for free could literally be the matter between life and death.

Community monitoring is not a panacea to curbing maternal deaths. Designing a health system that is steeped in equity and quality and combating the social determinants of health which drive maternal deaths is key.

But if we believe that we should have a say in the way our society, our communities and our country is run, then we should all be worried about the silence surrounding the deaths of 44,000 women from pregnancy-related causes every year. It is a gross injustice that needs to be set right.

References

Arya, N. (2013) Growth and development of tea industry in Assam. *International Journal of Scientific & Engineering Research* 4(7). Available at: https://www.ijser.org/paper/Growth-and-Development-of-Tea-Industry-in-Assam.html

Chaturvedi, S., Randive B., Diwan, V. et al. (2014) Quality of obstetric referral services in India's JSY cash transfer programme for institutional births: A study from Madhya Pradesh province'. *PLoS ONE* 9(5): e96773. Available at: https://journals.plos.org/plosone/article?id=10.1371/journal.pone.0096773

Government of Jharkhand (n.d.) *Bihar Scheduled Areas Regulation.* Available at: http://www.jharkhand.gov.in/documents/10179/54299/List%20Of%20Caste%20And%20SubCast%20under%20CNT%20ACT

Hazarika, L., Phukan, P., Sharma, A. and Das, N. K. (2017) Maternal mortality at a tertiary care teaching hospital in Dibrugarh district, Assam: a retrospective study. *International Journal of Community Medicine & Public Health* 4(9). Available at: https://www.ijcmph.com/index.php/ijcmph/article/view/1750

Intra Health International (2012) *Improving the Coverage and Quality of Village Health and Nutrition Days.* Available at: https://www.intrahealth.org/sites/ihweb/files/files/media/improving-the-coverage-and-quality-of-village-health-and-nutrition-days/VHND_UP_30_10_12.pdf

Kavle, J. A., Stoltzfus, R. J., Witter, F., et al. (2008) Association between anaemia during pregnancy and blood loss at and after delivery among women with vaginal births in Pemba Island, Zanzibar, Tanzania. *Journal of Health, Population & Nutrition* 26(2): 232–240. Available at: https://www.ncbi.nlm.nih.gov/pubmed/18686556

Mahanta, T. G., Mahanta, B. N., Gogoi, P., et al. (2015) Prevalence and determinants of anaemia and effect of different interventions amongst tea tribe adolescent girls living in Dibrugarh district of Assam. *Clinical Epidemiology & Global Health* 3(2), 85–93. Available at: https://www.ceghonline.com/article/S2213-3984(14)00042-6/fulltext/

National Institution for Transforming India (2018) Maternal mortality ratio (MMR). Government of India. Available at: https://niti.gov.in/content/maternal-mortality-ratio-mmr-100000-live-births

Office of the Registrar General and Census Commissioner (2011) Annual health survey 2010–11. Government of India. Available at: http://censusindia.gov.in/vital_statistics/AHSBulletins/files/05-Jharkhand_AHS_Bulletin__23x36_.pdf

Office of the Registrar General and Census Commissioner (2019) *District Census Hand Book – ASSAM,* Ministry of Home Affairs. Government of India. Available at: http://censusindia.gov.in/2011census/dchb/Assam.html

Randive, B., Diwan, V. and De Costa, A. (2013) India's conditional cash transfer programme (the JSY) to promote institutional birth: Is there an association between institutional birth proportion and maternal mortality?*PLoS ONE* 8(6): e67452. Available at: https://journals.plos.org/plosone/article?id=10.1371/journal.pone.0067452

Rao, S. (2017) *Do We Care? India's Health System.* New Delhi: Oxford University Press.

Sachdev, S. (2018) A matter of life and death: Surviving childbirth on Assam's tea plantations. Nazdeek. Available at: https://indd.adobe.com/view/aaf00c7a-8407-4ea0-982c-ca8b3555168a

Schudson, M. (2011) *The Good Citizen: A History of American Civic Life,* New York: The Free Press.

Scott, K. W., Phil, M. and Jha, A. K. (2014) Putting quality on the global health agenda. *The New England Journal of Medicine* 371:3–5. Available at: https://www.nejm.org/doi/full/10.1056/nejmp1402157

Sharma, J. B. and Shankar, M. (2010) Anemia in pregnancy. *Journal of International Medical Sciences Academy* 23(4): 253–260. Available at: http://medind.nic.in/jav/t10/i4/javt10i4p253.pdf

Sidney, K., Salazar, M., Marrone, G. et al. (2016) Out-of-pocket expenditures for childbirth in the context of the Janani Suraksha Yojana (JSY) cash transfer program to promote facility births: who pays and how much? Studies from Madhya Pradesh, India. *International Journal for Equity in Health*, 15:71. Available at: https://equityhealthj.biomedcentral.com/articles/10.1186/s12939-016-0362-4

Singh, P.K. (2018) *India has achieved groundbreaking success in reducing maternal mortality*. World Health Organisation. Available at: http://www.searo.who nt/mediacentre/features/2018/india-groundbreaking-sucess-reducing-maternal-mortality-rate/en/

Singh, S., Remez, L., Ram, Usha., et al. (2009) Barriers to Safe Motherhood in India. Guttmacher Institute. Available at: https://www.guttmacher.org/sites/default/files/report_pdf/safe-motherhood-india.pdf

Sri, S. B., and Khanna, R. (2014) *Dead Women Talking: A civil society report on maternal deaths in India,* Common Health & Jan Swasthya Abhiyan. Available at: http://www.commonhealth.in/Dead%20Women%20Talking%20full%20report%20final.pdf

United Nations Development Programme (2011) *Discussion Paper: A Social Determinants Approach to Maternal Health*. Available at: http://www.undp.org/content/dam/undp/library/Democratic%20Governance/Discussion%20Paper%20MaternalHealth.pdf

United Nations Secretary-General (2013) *Secretary-General's Remarks at High-Level Forum on Accelerating MDG-5*. United Nations. Available at: https://www.un.org/sg/en/content/sg/statement/2013-09-23/secretary-generals-remarks-high-level-forum-accelerating-mdg-5

World Health Organisation (2016) WHO recommendations on antenatal care for a positive pregnancy experience. United Nations. Available at: https://apps. who.int/iris/bitstream/handle/10665/250796/9789241549912-eng.pdf?sequence=1

Part II

Men over Women

CHAPTER 4

Without Consent*

Reproductive Rights under Attack

Patliputra Medical College and Hospital in the eastern state of Jharkhand is putrid. The squat toilets are overflowing and there's no water for patients to wash their hands. The hospital is teeming with people—so many that you literally have to step across pregnant women sprawled out on the grimy floors—to move through the corridors.

Birds have congregated on the inside of the hospital's roof to warm themselves from the harsh winter temperatures outside. The only evidence they exist—except for their occasional chirping—is their poo that is smeared across the floor and the barred windows. Several cows have gathered around the perimeter of the hospital too, occasionally making a run for the warmth inside, only to be whacked with whatever instrument—a walking stick, a scarf, a drink bottle—is sitting on the floor next to patients who are waiting to be seen by the doctors.

In the emergency room there are two almost lifeless women. They are lying next to one another on metal gurneys wrapped in red and

* Parts of this chapter have been published previously as Sophie Cousins, Botched sterilisation surgeries are killing Indian women. One woman wants to save them, *Elle*, 18 September 2019. Available at: https://www.elle.com/uk/life-and-culture/a23078460/botched-sterilisation-surgeries-killing-indian-women/

grey blankets pulled up to their chins. Both have IV drips attached to their wrists and their husbands by their side. They clutch their lower abdomens which, when they slowly push down their blankets, are revealed to be oversized and riddled with stitches.

A few days earlier the women had been sterilised at their local community health centre. Sterilisation, also known as tubal ligation, is a procedure in which the fallopian tubes are cut, tied or blocked to prevent future pregnancy.

The women live in a village on the outskirts of Dhanbad, Jharkhand's second largest city where Patliputra Medical College and Hospital is located. Dhanbad is a dusty, nondescript city with a constant flow of noisy, polluting trucks from the mines chugging through it. It's the height of winter and the near freezing temperatures mean that people wearing jumpers, beanies, socks and sandals are crowded on nearly every street corner burning rubbish and any other bit of waste they can find to get warm.

The women, Pouki Devi, 36, and Gudiya Devi, 30, had heard about a sterilisation camp from other women in their village. The camp was scheduled to run just a few minutes walk from their mud-brick homes. Both Pouki and Gudiya knew they didn't want to bear any more children—they'd both had four within a short time frame. Enough was enough, they thought. As gossip spread around the village about the camp, the women were excited as it was the first time they'd heard about a procedure that would, if done properly, ensure they wouldn't get pregnant again. Without knowing what the operation would entail and lacking knowledge about other possible contraceptive methods, they walked together on a brisk January Saturday morning to their local community healthcare centre.

Upon arriving, the first thing they noticed was how crowded it was. There was only one doctor present and the women worried they had come on the wrong day or to the wrong healthcare centre. There were dozens of women, just like them, lined up.

Clearly the message about the camp had gotten out.

Within just two hours the only doctor present had performed more than 30 sterilisations. A proper and hygienic sterilisation should take at least 20 minutes. The women were operated on and then tossed out like rags.

'There were so many people at the camp, the doctor rushed,' Pouki Devi, dressed in purple pyjamas, tells me.

During the procedure the doctor nicked both the women's bladders. As the doctor hastily tried to stitch their bladders back together they both fell unconscious.

They were both unconscious until they arrived at Patliputra Medical College and Hospital where they could receive proper medical attention.

'The doctor at the camp didn't utter a single word to us. He just referred us here. I don't know what has happened,' Gudiya's husband says angrily.

But sadly, Gudiya and Pouki's stories are not an anomaly—they are all too common, especially for poor rural women.

✳

For decades, sterilisation camps have been at the forefront of India's efforts to combat population growth.

The drive to sterilise India's burgeoning population began in the 1970s during a 21-month period known as the 'Emergency'. The Emergency was declared by then-Prime Minister Indira Gandhi in 1975, citing internal and external threats to the country including national security concerns, an ongoing drought and oil crisis, economic fragility, and ongoing political unrest.

Gandhi gave herself sweeping powers and as a result, the once thriving democracy was brought to a grinding halt. Elections and civil liberties were suspended; the notion of a 'free press' no longer existed and there was an unprecedented crackdown on those who opposed her governance.

Gandhi defended the Emergency on the grounds that she was trying to protect the State and Indian people, but it remains one of the most controversial periods in India's history, known as the 'The Dark Age of Indian Democracy'.

As Gandhi implemented welfare-style programmes and gave land to the poor who didn't own any, it came at a heavy cost. At the same time, Sanjay, Gandhi's son, began what has been described as a 'gruesome campaign' to sterilise the very people they were allegedly trying to help. The younger Gandhi was convinced population control was essential for India's economic development.

In some parts of the country poor men were offered plots of land in exchange for getting sterilised, or for encouraging others to do so. Village leaders and healthcare workers—like they still have today—had strict quotas to fill. But most of the time, land wasn't the prize. Instead, more often than not, some men were forcibly sterilised with police cordoning off villages and literally dragging them to the operating table. If police were not busy cordoning off villages, they were busy stopping buses and dragging men off to be sterilised. In some extreme cases, if men truthfully told police they had been sterilised, they were not believed and taken again for the procedure against their will (Mehta, 2012).

Between 1976 and 1977, 8.3 million men were sterilised (Chandra, 1987, p. 218). Sterilisation was no longer a choice—it was a mandate. Two thousand men died from botched operations and infections (Green, 2018).

India wasn't the only country that was determined to control the sub-continent's mushrooming population. Years before the Emergency, the United States had put pressure on Gandhi to pursue a more aggressive policy on population control. The US government was concerned that population growth was a threat to trade and its national security.

Population growth was also of major concern because at the time, in the 1960s, India faced a critical food shortage. There was a real fear of famine—a fear that history would repeat itself after the devastating famines that occurred under British colonial rule. This fear was spurred on by Stanford University professor Paul R. Ehrlich's alarmist book, *The Population Bomb*, which predicted hundreds of millions of people would die during the 1970s and 1980s. 'The streets seemed alive with people. People eating, people washing, people sleeping.

People visiting, people arguing and screaming. People thrust their hands through the taxi window, begging,' he wrote about his trip to India (1968, p. 15). 'People defecating and urinating. People clinging to buses. People herding animals. People, people, people, people. Since that night, I've known the horror of overpopulation. The battle to feed humanity is over, and humanity is lost' (1968, p. 15).

The push to sterilise became so great that in 1965, then-American President Lyndon Johnson refused to provide food aid to India until it agreed to incentivise sterilisation. The preordained drive to sterilise was supported by loans from the World Bank, different United Nations agencies and the Swedish International Development Authority. In 1952, the Indian government initiated what by the 1960s would become the world's largest state-sponsored family planning programme. While the programme initially focused on women, it soon shifted to men, spurred on by social scientists who argued the government needed to target men for economic reasons. 'Having reframed family planning as a cognitive phenomenon involving a degree of calculation and forethought, scientists continually referred to Indian men's ostensibly greater contributions to economic decision-making and capacity for calculative reasoning,' Savina Balasubramanian, a political sociologist, argues (2018, p. 46). In 1962, sociologist Donald Bogue argued that there was 'very little cultural or sociological basis to support a program in which the wife takes the lead in gaining information about family planning and convinces an unwilling or disinterested husband ... Making the male the primary target for educational and motivational efforts conforms to the realities of the "power structure" within the Indian family' (Bogue, 1962, p. 512).

But the decision to put the onus on men for family planning came to a standstill following the coercive targeting of millions of men to undergo vasectomies during the Emergency period. After 1977, state governments and political parties refocused family planning agendas. Men were no longer the target.

And so decades on, sterilisation remains at the core of India's family planning policy. But instead of focusing on men, the onus is now on women—women who are less likely to protest and who, in many parts of the country, have little, if any, agency over their own bodies. Sterilisation is cheap, effective and easily solves the challenges of providing other methods of contraception in rural and remote areas.

Unlike China, which until recently had a one-child policy to slow population growth, India's government offers cash incentives to women and men who opt for permanent sterilisation.

Depending on where they live, women and men are given a cash incentive of between ₹1400 (US$19.60) to ₹3000 (US$41.90) (Dhar, 2015).

It's not only the women and men who undergo the procedure who are compensated.

Community healthcare workers, known as Accredited Social Health Activists (ASHAs), are remunerated for being 'motivators'. In other words an ASHA worker will be rewarded if she brings a woman to be sterilised—which in almost all cases is a woman—and a doctor will also be given a bonus for each woman he or she operates on. If sterilisations happen at private facilities or non-government organisations, they are also compensated.

These workers are not just driven by financial incentives (they do not receive a salary) but also by pressure to reach informal monthly sterilisation 'targets' by which the government measures progress, regardless of the circumstances in which the operation takes place. While national targets for sterilisation were officially eliminated 20 years ago, the practice continues today at some state and district levels. Healthcare workers know if they do not meet these unofficial targets they could face salary cuts or dismissal.

In 2016, the government launched 'Mission Parivar Vikas', a programme to specifically target the designated 145 'high fertility districts' in seven states across the country which constitute 44 per cent of the country's population. The aim of the programme is to reduce the fertility level in these areas from 3.0 to 2.1 by 2025 (Press Information Bureau, 2016). Women who live in any of the designated 145 'high fertility districts' like the tribal areas of Jharkhand are offered more money to undergo sterilisation.

But this approach, like the Emergency period, disproportionately focuses on the rural poor and uneducated—those who are blamed for India's burgeoning population and thus its trials and tribulations from poverty to hunger.

As a result, every year approximately four million women undergo sterilisation in India, more than in anywhere else in the world. But many come away with a lot more than not being able to bear children anymore.

Informal sterilisation targets and cash incentives for healthcare workers have created an environment where mass operations carried out in unsafe conditions are the norm, often with deadly consequences. Moreover, it has created an environment where women are treated like cattle, brought by the dozens into camps, often without understanding what they have just consented to.

∗

One brisk Saturday night in the village of Kaparfora in the northern state of Bihar, one of India's poorest states, a doctor sterilised 53 women in two hours under the supervision of a local NGO. It was early 2012 and the doctor performed the procedure on school desks in the pitch dark, the only source of light being a torchlight that an assistant held over the women's bodies. Throughout the course of the evening the doctor never changed his gloves, there was no running water and the medicines he used were past their use-by-dates. The procedures were carried out on dirty, dusty school desks that were never disinfected. After he was finished, the doctor left the school ignoring the screams of women lying on the classroom floor. Three had been left bleeding profusely; another had been sterilised while being three months pregnant.

The following year in Malda, a district in West Bengal, almost 100 unconscious rural women were dumped in an open field after being sterilised at a camp at a healthcare centre. They were thrown in the field to recover from their operations because there was no room for them at the centre.

And just over a year later, in November 2014, a doctor and his assistant performed 140 sterilisations on women in two different camps in Bilaspur, a city in the central Indian state of Chhattisgarh. Months earlier the doctor had received an award from the Chhattisgarh government for conducting over 50,000 sterilisations—an achievement deemed worthy of public praise. Two days after the camps eight women died. A few days later another five died. Seventy were hospitalised with severe complications. It was revealed that the doctor had performed 83 of the sterilisations in just six hours, breaching government guidelines that stipulate surgeons to perform no more than 30 sterilisations per day. While the exact cause of the women's deaths remains unknown, post-mortem investigations found they died either from the repeated use of unsterilised, dirty equipment or contaminated medicines—or both (Jan Swasthya Abhiyan et al., 2014).

Widespread national and international attention and condemnation of the three tragedies brought the issue of sterilisation again back into the public sphere with women's health activists and family members asking: Why are our women dying during sterilisation? Where are the other contraceptive methods? Who is going to be held accountable for the atrocities that are being committed?

Accountability was something that the Supreme Court had tried to address back in 2007. The disasters of 2012, 2013 and 2014 weren't something new—for years stories of women being sterilised without consent, in unsafe, unhygienic conditions, by drunk doctors, even by bicycle pumps because doctors didn't have up-to-date equipment—had plagued almost every state across the country. Some garnered local, national and international attention, but many more went ignored.

Following a petition regarding concerns that women going for sterilisation lacked counselling or informed consent, pre-and post-operative care and faced coercion and cruelty, in 2007 the Supreme Court ruled that the central government was responsible for maintaining standards in sterilisation procedures (Supreme Court of India, 2007). The Court also asked state governments—who are responsible for health—to introduce quality assurance commissions to ensure high standards in clinics, underscoring the desperate need for required informed consent, punitive actions for violations and compensation for victims. But more than a decade on, such bodies have not been functioning as envisioned. And according to the latest government figures, between 2012 and 2016, 537 women lost their lives to sterilisation, some as young as 18 years old (Bhuyan, 2018). The women who have suffered from botched operations likely number in thousands, though the precise number is unknown.

'Sometimes we make mistakes,' Nabakanta Sharma, a gynaecologist and obstetrician in the north-eastern state of Manipur, tells me. 'I have sterilised between 50,000 and 70,000 women. I've actually stopped counting. Sometimes I have done 100 plus operations in a day. The standard isn't good.'

✳

One woman couldn't shake the 2012 incident in Bihar where 53 women had been sterilised by one doctor in two hours. She was unable to get the voices of wailing women out of her head. She knew she had to do something.

A native of Bihar, Devika Biswas, is an indefatigable women's health activist living in the eastern state of Jharkhand. A month after the incident, Biswas went back to her home state on a fact-finding mission. She wanted to know why and how it had all gone so terribly wrong and who—if anyone—was being held accountable. She was to report her findings to the National Alliance for Maternal Health and the Human Rights and Healthwatch Forum, two local organisations that monitor reproductive violations against women in the most far-flung areas of India. When she arrived home she was lost for words, aghast at what she heard.

She recalls what the woman who had been operated on while being pregnant told her: 'For the government, people like me, life has no meaning so they can do anything with us.'

Biswas was devastated. Devastated that her own people were being treated like this. Her devastation was only amplified by the realisation that any number of the young women she met and interviewed could have been her daughter.

With help from lawyers in New Delhi, Biswas filed a petition to the Supreme Court based on her findings. After a four year battle with the government, in September 2016, the court ordered the government to shut down sterilisation camps across the country within three years. The camps, the court judgement said, infringe on the 'reproductive freedoms of the most vulnerable groups of society whose economic and social conditions leave them with no meaningful choice ... and render them the easiest targets of coercion' (Social Protection and Human Rights, 2016).

'It is time that women and men are treated with respect and dignity and not as mere statistics in the sterilisation programme,' it further read.

The verdict issued several critical directives, including that governments no longer stipulate fixed targets for sterilisation so healthcare workers and others do not compel or force women to undergo such operations; to increase compensations for sterilisation deaths and botched operations; and to mandatorily explain to patients, in his or her language, the impact and consequence of the procedure.

While women will still be able to undergo sterilisation, camps run by state governments or local NGOs will be banned.

The verdict was hailed as a significant step in the right direction for women's sexual and reproductive health and rights. Women's health activists around the country celebrated, believing that finally the moment had arrived for the government to take the onus off women for family planning, and in doing so provide a wider range of contraception, available to all.

But at the time of writing, just nine months before the September 2019 deadline, camps in many parts of the country continue to thrive in the same way. Many state governments still unofficially enforce targets for sterilisation.

'It's actually naïve to imagine that orders passed by the Supreme Court would lead to significantly changed practices on the ground,' Jashodhara Dasgupta, head of the National Foundation for India and founder of SAHAYOG, a NGO which works on maternal health and rights, tells me.

And perhaps she's right.

One major concern is that there is no accountability or monitoring mechanism in place to observe if governments have stopped the camps or have stopped its target-based approach to sterilisation.

'There is no positive light from the field. Governments are still continuing the target approach,' Sarita Barpanda, from Human Rights Law Network, which played an integral role in bringing Biswas's case before the court, tells me. 'Why is it so important for men and women to be sterilised? It's almost like it has been seeped into people's minds that population explosion is the one reason why India is facing the majority [of] its problems.'

SAHAYOG has been monitoring media reports about sterilisation deaths and botched operations since the judgement in 2016. There have been too many incidents to name and sadly the reported ones—those that are in the public domain—are just the tip of the iceberg.

Women's health activists, including Biswas, fear that government efforts to redefine camps—by calling them something else on paper—will mean they will continue to flourish.

'They (state governments) are still doing camps but without saying it's a camp so on paper it becomes a "health day",' she tells me.

'Moving forward there will be fixed dates, which means a doctor will allocate a day a week for sterilisation so anyone who wants to come on the day, the operating theatre will be ready.'

In other words, Biswas worries that mass operations will continue to thrive. She also worries that as long as state governments remunerate healthcare workers for the procedure, they will continue to coerce women into the procedure.

Her fear is something that keeps Dasgupta awake at night. Both want the incentive system for sterilisation to be abolished immediately.

'If you convince someone for sterilisation, this is hugely problematic,' Dasgupta tells me at her new office in New Delhi.

✳

Back at Patliputra Medical College and Hospital, Biswas is busily scribbling down notes in her battered notebook. At one point she runs out of space to take any more notes and starts dictating to me. I scribble down her observations as quickly as my hand can move before she moves on to interview Pouki and Gudiya about their botched operations. After getting a call early this morning about a camp that had gone terribly wrong, Biswas and I travelled several hours to Dhanbad so she could undertake another fact-finding mission. It's something she's gotten all too used to. She wants to hold the government to account for the botched operations and at the very least she wants the women to be reimbursed for the medical costs they've incurred.

'I will keep all your paperwork. I will report it to the government of Jharkhand. You should be paid for your hospitalisation,' she tells the women.

They nod, sincerely appreciating Biswas's efforts.

Biswas turns to me and shakes her head.

'No one monitors the sterilisation camps because no one thinks anyone will come and ask about them,' she says.

If India is going to finally end its dark history with sterilisation it will need to put strict monitoring and accountability mechanisms in place to ensure the Supreme Court judgement is respected.

Moreover, a wide range of contraceptive methods from the pill to the injectable need to be available for women in an enabling and friendly environment. In order for women to access such methods, they must be empowered to make informed choices; they must have agency over their own bodies. After all, choice is at the very heart of this issue. But as Poonam Muttreja, executive director of the Population Foundation of India stresses, this is not just about women. It's about men too.

'Family planning is not a women's issue. It should be a people's issue. Sex happens between two people. A man has to take just as much responsibility as a woman and in fact, more, because women don't have agency. Until women get equality, family planning should be a man's responsibility,' she says.

∗

Outside, the mid-morning heat radiating off the orange yolk sun is already stifling. The dry heat of New Delhi is the type of heat that exhausts you to your bone, made all the worse by a thick layer of pollution that feels like it is entering your bloodstream like lava.

The maternity ward inside the hospital attached to Jamia Hamdard University in southern Delhi is long, narrow and sparse. A dozen or so metal gurneys are all occupied and a handful of ceiling fans are spinning at their full capacity, trying desperately to circulate some cool air. But the fans are so decrepit that they sound like they're about to fall off their rusty hinges.

Women are curled up on their sides, their arms embracing the tiny babies they've recently given life to. Their mothers and mothers-in-law crowd around the beds partaking in the celebrations. But not all women are here to give birth.

Vidya arrived at the hospital with her mother yesterday.[1] She's 18, two months pregnant and unmarried—a huge taboo in India. She's not here for a check-up, though, she's here for an abortion. Though if she had a choice, she would not be here to terminate her pregnancy.

India legalised abortion in 1971 when it passed the Medical Termination of Pregnancy (MTP) Act. The procedure is allowed if a woman or her baby's physical or mental health is under threat. The law includes women under 18 as long as they have their guardian's consent, and women made pregnant by rape. A woman doesn't need the consent of her husband and can legally terminate at up to 20 weeks' gestation (discussions are ongoing to extend this to 24 weeks).

---

[1] Part of this story has been published previously in Sophie Cousins, Abortion, contraception, pregnancy: how women's bodies became a battlezone, *Mosaic Science*, 12 September 2017. Available at: https://mosaicscience.com/story/contraception-abortion-pregnancy-womens-rights-US-India/

And in a society obsessed with marriage, one clause is specifically reserved for married women only: abortion because of contraceptive failure.

But in many cases like Vidya's, nurses and doctors ignore the fact she is not married and perform the procedure anyway, knowing full well that if it doesn't happen here, it'll happen elsewhere and perhaps unsafely.

Wearing an oversized navy jumper, Vidya lies on her bed, facing away from her mother. She occasionally rubs her tummy like it's a reminder to her mother that she is being forced to do something she doesn't want to do.

'We do not agree with continuing this pregnancy,' her mother tells me. 'She has brought great shame on the family.' I ask Vidya if she will continue to see her boyfriend, who, like her, is in XI standard—the second-to-last year of school. Her mother doesn't give her daughter an opportunity to answer and instead tells me: 'I will talk to him and his family also and after some time, after he completes his study, she will agree to do the marriage.'

Vidya looks vacantly at the ceiling fan above her, her fate already sealed.

'Yes, I plan for marriage at the end of the year.'

✳

On paper, India's MTP Act is liberal and stands in stark contrast to many countries around the world where abortion, in the face of growing right-wing populism, has become even more of a politicised and polarising issue.

But despite abortion being legal in India and with little opposition against it, the reality on the ground paints a very different story.

Every day close to eight women die from unsafe abortion in India (Singh et al., 2018b). The deaths account for nine per cent of the estimated 44,000 maternal deaths every year across the country (Doskoch, 2014).

Abortion incidence is an important indicator of women's need to access safe abortion services and of their unmet need for contraception. The government has a responsibility to report reliable abortion and unintended pregnancy figures so they can be used to guide policy. It's no surprise then that the government's own figures on abortion incidence across the country are significantly lower than independent estimations. For the last 15 years, the Ministry of Health and Family Welfare has recorded between 621,000 and 770,000 abortions each year (Singh et al., 2018a).

But according to the first national study of the incidence of abortion and unintended pregnancy in India, an estimated 15.6 million abortions were performed in 2015 (Singh et al., 2018a).

The study found 3.4 million abortions were obtained in health facilities, 11.5 million abortions were medical abortions done outside of health facilities and 0.8 million abortions were done outside of health facilities through 'other methods that were probably unsafe' (Singh et al., 2018a).

So why are so many women seeking abortions outside the healthcare system when they can—in theory—legally go to their nearest primary healthcare centre or hospital for the procedure?

Millions of women and girls face structural, institutional and cultural barriers that prevent them from accessing abortion services.

Unsafe abortion is defined by the World Health Organisation as 'a procedure for terminating an unwanted pregnancy either by persons lacking the necessary skills or in an environment lacking minimal medical standards or both' (2012).

While the reasons why women die from abortion have changed over time, the number of women dying every year in India remains stagnant, despite medical advancements that have enabled the procedure to be easier and safer.

Deaths from unsafe abortion have historically been driven by traditional providers, also known as quacks, who, without any medical training, give women herbal medicines and roots, or shove sticks or other items inside women to induce abortion. Such methods, while still common, have significantly declined in recent years.

Instead, unsafe abortion in India is commonly carried out by women themselves by taking unapproved and ineffective drugs or by taking highly efficacious, safe and approved drugs, as per a method known as medical abortion, incorrectly. The women are of course not at fault—ignorant pharmacists are doing wrong by women and are putting their lives at risk.

Medical abortion—that is, the use of misoprostol and mifepristone which work together to end pregnancy within the first ten weeks—is a safe and proven method of abortion. It is far safer than other precarious methods which have previously dominated the landscape.

✳

The 2015 Health Facilities Survey, a survey of abortion incidence and unintended pregnancy in six Indian states (Assam, Bihar, Gujarat, Madhya Pradesh, Tamil Nadu and Uttar Pradesh) found that only a minority of abortions occurring in each state are actually carried out at health facilities (Singh et al., 2018b).

For example, only 11 per cent of the estimated 3.2 million abortions in Uttar Pradesh every year occur in health facilities. Of those that do occur in health facilities, the majority are provided by the private sector (Singh et al., 2018b).

According to guidelines issued by the Ministry of Health and Family Welfare (MoHFW), all public sector facilities at the primary health centre level and higher are allowed to provide induced abortion, as long as they have a certificated provider on staff (2010).

Primary health centres (PHCs) are the cornerstone of the rural healthcare system—a system that hundreds of millions, particularly the poor, rely on for free care. But few primary health centres offer abortion services.

For example, in Bihar, only five per cent of primary health centres (PHCs) offer abortion services (Singh et al., 2018b). But it's not only PHCs that are failing to provide care. Community health centres (CHCs) which act as referral centres for PHCs and hospitals should also have the trained staff and equipment to provide abortion. But they too are failing women.

For example, in Uttar Pradesh, India's most populous state, only 27 per cent of hospitals, CHCs and other urban public facilities provide abortion services (Singh et al., 2018b).

While the Health Facilities Survey only included six states, those states are home to 45 per cent of India's women of reproductive age and likely give an accurate representation of what is going on throughout the country.

So what has gone so terribly wrong? Why are so few public health facilities offering abortion services? A lack of trained staff, equipment and staff shortages, failure to provide confidential care, healthcare worker stigma, misconceptions about the law, and a lack of priority given to women in the healthcare system are some reasons why.

Another major barrier is the Pre-Conception and Pre-Natal Diagnostics Techniques (PCPNDT) Act, discussed in chapter one, which prohibits the misuse of prenatal diagnostic tests for sex determination.

In recent years the government has used the media to disseminate messages around the consequences of the continued and widespread use of ultrasounds for sex determination. As a result, more and more doctors are hesitant to provide abortion services because of real and perceived crackdowns by authorities on healthcare providers who carry out sex-selective abortions. This, however, has had a grave impact on the women who want to terminate their pregnancies for legal reasons.

In addition to institutional barriers, there are deep-seated cultural and structural barriers that also work to restrict or prevent women from accessing safe abortion. Such barriers are similar to the barriers that prevent women from using contraception in the first place.

For those who are able to access abortion services, although the procedure is technically free of charge at public facilities, women incur direct costs such as paying for medicines and anesthesia and indirect costs such as transportation and loss of earnings for the day. Such costs can prevent women from physically accessing services or can force families into debt.

But as countless public health facilities fail to even offer abortion services, many women have no option but to turn to the private sector for the procedure—an industry driven by the blind pursuit of money instead of quality care.

'It is sad in a country where abortion is legal that women can't afford to go to a facility,' Vinoj Manning, executive director of Ipas India, a non-governmental organisation focused on preventing deaths from unsafe abortion, says.

But even when safe services are available and women are aware that such services exist, stigma surrounding abortion hugely impacts health-seeking behaviour. For young women, fear of stigma can be so great that many choose to continue their unintended pregnancy for fear of retaliation from family members or seek out underground abortion services (Sebastian et al., 2014).

Inevitably for a woman to be able to seek out an abortion, she must know that it is legal. But less than 20 per cent of Indian women know that abortion is legal (V. Manning, personal communication). Even among those who are aware the procedure is legal, many mistakenly believe that a husband's consent is required.

Another major barrier is gender inequality: a woman's lack of agency and her inability to make decisions about her own body.

'Women do not have the authority or the opportunity to make decisions about any aspect of their life and childbearing seems to be a decision which is not a decision,' Poonam Muttreja, from the Population Foundation of India, says.

Driven by the notion of shame and fear, almost half of women seeking an abortion don't tell their husbands (P. Muttreja, personal communication). As a result, Muttreja believes that for every woman who dies from abortion, there are 20 women who 'live life dying' through serious morbidities because of how unsafe abortions are carried out.

'[Women] don't want their husbands to know they're getting an abortion because often abortion is a proxy for contraception. Women are not expected to use contraceptives [but] abortion would be a much worse offence,' she says.

All these factors combined have led to a thriving over-the-counter use of medical abortion.

In 2002, India approved registered medical practitioners to provide medical abortion in accredited facilities for women up to seven weeks' gestation. In 2003 it extended the law to allow these providers to prescribe the drugs in other settings, meaning that women could get the pills over-the-counter with a prescription.

The idea was that by enabling women to purchase the pills over-the-counter with a prescription it would deter them from seeking unsafe abortions by quacks or uncertified abortion providers.

Countries around the world have demonstrated that medical abortion is a safe and highly effective method for women to do alone. The benefits, particularly the privacy and discretion it affords women, cannot be underestimated. It enables women to overcome some of the key barriers that prevent them from going to a hospital such as lack of accessibility, stigma and concerns around privacy and confidentiality.

Research shows that in India over 85 per cent of sales of misoprostol and mifepristone take place without a prescription (Powell-Jackson, 2015).

Failing to ask women for a prescription for medical abortion is not necessarily a bad thing because it removes some of the barriers that prevent women from seeking out a doctor to write one. What, however, is detrimental to women is that pharmacists are failing in their duties to inform women how to take the pills correctly.

Pharmacists are routinely failing to ask women critical questions such as when their last period occurred (Powell-Jackson, 2015). Moreover, they are failing to explain to women how and when to take the pills and often resort to giving traditional medicines instead (Powell-Jackson, 2015).

Giving women traditional or alternative medicines can have devastating consequences and so can giving women incorrect inform-ation about how to take misoprostol and mifepristone. Both can lead to incomplete abortion, which can lead to severe complications including severe bleeding and death.

'We know that women are practising abortion alone, we know that, yet we do not make all the information available,' Muttreja says.

'I am supportive of women having access [to medical abortion] but I'm not supportive of the fact we are not telling women how they should use it. Pharmacies should be able to explain to women how to do it. But women are so dispensable that we just experiment with them.'

A recent study in the central Indian state of Madhya Pradesh found that 80 per cent of chemists gave no advice or incorrect advice on the gestational limit for medical abortion and about two-thirds gave incorrect information on administering the two-pill regimen (Powell-Jackson, 2015). It is no surprise then that women continue to die from unsafe abortion or face serious morbidities when they do not receive accurate information on how to carry out a safe method of abortion.

But as demand for its availability shows no sign of waning, in recent years some policy-makers believe it would be best to restrict women's access to it. The change in attitude has been driven by the perceived misuse of misoprostol and mifepristone and the skewed sex ratio that shows no sign of rectifying itself. In some states this belief has turned into action.

'I'm just a regular abortion provider but I believe in reproductive rights and the right to abort for all women is a non-negotiable. We need to ensure there are no barriers in accessing abortion,' Dr Jaydeep Tank, a gynecologist practising in Mumbai, says.

'Unfortunately the perception that medical abortion tablets are abused is leading policy-makers to restrict their use. The real concern is that this will deprive women of a method that is safe.'

The southern state of Maharashtra is one state that is working to restrict women's access to medical abortion. When the 2011 Census results were released, policy-makers were confronted with the reality that the skewed sex ratio wasn't reducing.

Believing that women were to blame—that they were misusing medical abortion to abort the girls they didn't want—the state moved to implement stronger abortion regulations. Investigations found that some chemists and clinics had stopped stocking and dispensing medical abortion drugs which not only severely restricted women's access to the drugs over-the-counter but also restricted certified abortion providers' access to them (Iyer, 2013). In 2012, a study of more than 200 chemists in Maharashtra found that medical abortion pills were only available in 10 per cent of chemists while 58 per cent reported they stopped stocking the drugs after the government began enforcing new regulations (Singh et al., 2018b).

The current extent of the unavailability of medical abortion in Maharashtra and beyond is unknown; there are no published studies to understand the magnitude of the problem.

Ultimately millions of women across India will continue to seek abortions not only because contraceptive methods fail, but because women have an unmet need for contraception. Restricting women's access to medical abortion sets a dangerous precedent and will only result in more women seeking potentially deadly underground unsafe abortions.

✳

It's June 2017 and the rains have already arrived in the north-eastern Indian state of Manipur. Apple-green rice paddies, wild, rolling hills and low-lying grey clouds surround Imphal, the state's capital. Manipur, like the seven other states of the north-east, is separated from the mainland by Bangladesh. Though part of India, the impact of separation from the mainland is conspicuous. Imphal feels isolated, like it's stuck in time as the rest of India continues to develop at a rapid speed. It feels familiar to neighbouring Myanmar and Nepal—from the dust-lined streets to chicken momos steaming in oversized metal pots in shop fronts.

The Regional Institute of Medical Sciences (RIMS)—a government hospital in western Imphal—is bustling. The one-level hospital is filled with families who have travelled hundreds of kilometres to see a doctor. Many have been waiting for days to see a doctor and are camped along the hospital's corridors, their belongings in tow.

The maternity ward is sprawled across three rooms. It's teeming with people, young and old, and tears of joy.

Two days ago, 21-year-old Sanathoi travelled 17 kilometres from her village to give birth to her first child. Sanathoi has a round, delicate face and almond eyes and ties her shiny black hair in a low bun. Unlike her mother who gave birth to all her ten children at home, Sanathoi decided to give birth in a facility.[2]

Sanathoi says that her baby was unplanned.

'I don't know how to prevent pregnancy,' she tells me, cradling her baby in her arms.

'I don't plan to use family planning. I don't know of any methods. I think I'll be pressured to have another baby. I can't even think about it.'

Sanathoi is one of a growing number of women in Manipur who have an unmet need for contraception—women who want to delay or stop childbearing but who are not using any method of contraception. Over the last decade, according to the latest National Family Health Survey, the unmet need for contraception in the north-eastern state has doubled from 16 per cent in 2005 to 30 per cent in 2015 (International Institute for Population Sciences, 2017). At the same time, the use of modern contraceptives—such as the pill, condoms, IUDs and sterilisation—has almost halved from 24 per cent to 13 per cent (International Institute for Population Sciences, 2017). Reasons for the significant change is unclear. But what is clear is that

---

[2] Part of this story has been published previously in Sophie Cousins, Abortion, contraception, pregnancy: how women's bodies became a battlezone, *Mosaic Science*, 12 September 2017. Available at: https://mosaicscience.com/story/contraception-abortion-pregnancy-womens-rights-US-India/

not a single community health worker otherwise known as Accredited Social Health Activists (ASHAs)—who are meant to be present in every village across India to advise and educate on family planning—has visited Sanathoi's village to teach women about contraception.

Across India, almost one in seven married women aged 15–49 don't want to get pregnant at the moment but are not using contraception (International Institute for Population Sciences, 2017). Of the 48 per cent of women who are using modern contraception, just over four per cent rely on the pill, 1.5 per cent on IUDs and 5.6 per cent on condoms (International Institute for Population Sciences, 2017). Female sterilisation makes up 86 per cent of modern contraceptive use.

The barriers that prevent women from accessing contraception are inevitably similar to the factors that restrict women's access to abortion, including institutional barriers such as a lack of trained healthcare providers, contraceptive stock-outs, lack of contraceptive choice and prohibitive costs. And then there are the cultural and structural barriers including stigma, a lack of education and women's agency, men's reluctance to take responsibility for family planning, and traditional norms that dictate that a woman's primary duty is to reproduce.

'As soon as women get married they're expected to give proof of their fertility. Women cannot negotiate contraception. It's something they have to keep to themselves because even if a woman suggests her husband to wear a condom, she's seen as promiscuous,' Muttreja tells me.

In addition to the barriers mentioned, there's another major obstacle: rumours. The most widespread rumour is that male sterilisation, otherwise known as a vasectomy, will reduce men's libidos and make sex less pleasurable.

The latest data shows that male sterilisation has decreased from one per cent to 0.3 per cent in the last decade (International Institute for Population Sciences, 2017). While some point to India's dark history of coerced male sterilisation as a reason for its unpopularity, many more men seem worried about the mistaken belief that a vasectomy will make sex less pleasurable and will make them weak. Whatever the source of the rumours, they only work to propagate the message that family planning is a woman's issue and thus her responsibility.

Recognising the embarrassingly low uptake of vasectomy, the government plans to increase the proportion of male sterilisation from less than one per cent to at least 30 per cent (National Health Policy, 2017). The policy, however, neglects to specify how it will achieve this goal and within what time frame.

But the problem isn't just sterilisation. Condoms are also shrouded in myths and men have reported problems buying them because of perceived stigma (Donta, Begum and Naik, 2014).

At the very heart of the issue is getting men to take responsibility for family planning; getting them to recognise that they too should be a part of it.

But as long as women do not have access to a wide range of contraceptive methods, financial incentives for everyone involved with sterilisation remains in place and vasectomy is snubbed, female sterilisation will continue to be the most popular contraceptive method.

'The tragedy is that 77 per cent of women that undergo sterilisation have never experienced family planning ever in [their] lives which shows that they do not have access to temporary methods of contraception,' Muttreja tells me.

'When you don't have choice and when the health worker doesn't give you a choice of [different contraceptive methods], what is it? It is coercion.'

The most concrete way of empowering a woman is enabling her to control her fertility.

But as long as women's bodies are used as reproducing machines, like factory-farmed chickens for their eggs, realising women's reproductive health rights seems more like a distant dream than a reality.

References

Balasubramanian, S. (2018) Motivating men: Social science and the regulation of men's reproduction in postwar India. *Sage Journals* 32(1): 34–58. Available at: https://journals.sagepub.com/doi/10.1177/0891243217743221

Bhuyan, A. (2018) Chhattisgarh's sterilisation deaths have changed nothing for family planning burden on women. *The Wire*, 13 January 2018. Available at: https://thewire.in/health/sterilization-family-planning-women-burden

Bogue, D. J. (1962) Some tentative recommendations for a 'sociologically correct' family planning communication and motivation program in India, in Kiser, C. V. (ed.). *Research in Family Planning,* New Jersey, Princeton: Princeton University Press.

Chandra, S. K. (1987) *Family Planning Programme in India: Its Impact in Rural And Urban Areas- 1970–1980.* Delhi: Mittal Publications.

Dhar, A. (2015) Gendered approach to sterilization. *The Hindu*, 1 January 2015. Available at: https://www.thehindu.com/sci-tech/health/policy-and-issues/gendered-approach-to-sterilisation/article6742284.ece

Donta, B., Begum, S. and Naik, D. D. (2014) Acceptability of male condom: An Indian scenario. *Indian Journal of Medical Research* 140(7):152–156. Available at: http://www.ijmr.org.in/article.asp?issn=0971-5916;year=2014;volume=140;issue=7;spage=152;epage=156;aulast=Donta

Doskoch, P. (2014) Maternal mortality is declining, but not enough to meet Millennium Development Goal 5. *International Perspectives on Sexual And Reproductive Health* 40(2): 100–101. Available at: https://www.guttmacher.org/journals/ipsrh/2014/07/maternal-mortality-declining-not-enough-meet-millennium-development-goal-5

Ehrlich, P. R. (1968) *The Population Bomb.* Sierra Club/Ballantine Books.

Green, H. H. (2018) Why is the burden of sterilisation on women in India? The answer lies in the Emergency Era. *Scroll*, 10 October 2018. Available at: https://scroll.in/article/896925/why-is-the-burden-of-sterilisation-on-women-in-india-the-answer-lies-in-the-emergency-era

International Institute for Population Sciences (2017) *National Family Health Survey-4 (2015–2016).* Available at: http://rchiips.org/nfhs/factsheet_NFHS-4.shtml

Iyer, M. (2013) State driving abortion pills out of the market. *Times of India*, 25 April 2013. Available at: https://timesofindia.indiatimes.com/city/mumbai/State-driving-abortion-pills-out-of-market/articleshow/19718182.cms

Jan Swasthya Abhiyan et al. (2014) *Camp of Wrongs: The Mourning Afterwards.* Available at: http://feministlawarchives.pldindia.org/wp-content/uploads/Camp-of-Wrongs-the-mourning-afterwards-A-fact-finding-report-on-sterilisation-deaths-in-Bilaspur-by-SAMA-2014.pdf

Ministry of Health and Family Welfare (2010) *Comprehensive Abortion Care: Training and Service Delivery Guidelines,* Government of India. Available at: http://www.nhm.gov.in/images/pdf/programmes/maternal-health/guidelines/abortion_care_training.pdf

Mehta, V. (2012) *The Sanjay Story: From Anand Bhavan To Amethi.* India: HarperCollins.

Powell-Jackson, T., Acharya, R., Filippi, V. et al. (2015) Delivering medical abortion at scale: A study of the retail market for medical abortion in Madhya Pradesh, India. *PLoS One,* 10(*3*): e0120637. Available at: https://journals.plos.org/plosone/article?id=10.1371/journal.pone.0120637

Press Information Bureau (2016) Health Ministry to launch 'Mission Parivar Vikas' in 145 high focus districts for improved family planning services. Ministry of Health and Family Welfare, Government of India. Available at: http://pib.nic.in/newsite/PrintRelease.aspx?relid=151049

Sebastian, M. P., Khan, M. E. and Sebastian, D. (2013) *Unintended Pregnancy and Abortion in India with Focus on Bihar, Madhya Pradesh and Odisha,* New Delhi, India: Population Council. Available at: https://www.popcouncil.org/uploads/pdfs/2014STEPUP_IndiaCountryProfile.pdf

Singh, S., Shekhar, C., Acharya, R. et al. (2018a) The incidence of abortion and unintended pregnancy in India, 2015. *The Lancet Global Health* 6 (*1*): 111–120.

Singh, S., Hussain, R., Shekhar, C. et al. (2018b) *Abortion and Unintended Pregnancy in Six Indian States: Findings and Implications for Policies and Programs.* New York: Guttmacher Institute. Available at: https://www.guttmacher.org/report/abortion-unintended-pregnancy-six-states-india

Social Protection and Human Rights (2016) Sexual and reproductive health and rights in India. Available at: https://socialprotection-humanrights.org/legaldep/sexual-reproductive-health-rights-india/

Supreme Court of India (2007) Record of Proceedings, Writ Petition (Civil) No. 209/2003. Available at: https://www.escr-net.org/sites/default/files/SC_Order_RAMAKANT%20RAI_%20Sterilisation.pdf

World Health Organisation (2012) Unsafe abortion incidence and mortality - Global and regional levels in 2008 and trends. United Nations. Available at: https://www.who.int/reproductivehealth/publications/unsafe_abortion/rhr_12_01/en/

CHAPTER 5

Fighting Stigma
HIV and Tuberculosis

In 2007, 17-year-old Nandita Venkatesan could barely contain her excitement at beginning her undergraduate studies at Ramnarain Ruia College in Mumbai. She was thrilled to have been accepted into one of the country's most prestigious colleges and to leave her school years behind.

But just one month into her studies, Nandita began experiencing severe lower abdominal pain, frequent bouts of vomiting, extreme nausea, fever, and loss of appetite.

It was the monsoon season in Mumbai, and like every year, heavy rains lashed the city, flooding homes, businesses and roads. While the rains arrive like clockwork every year, 2007 was a particularly bad year. The country's financial capital came to a grinding halt as water levels rose to knee level in the streets, forcing train services and flights to be cancelled. Made worse by poor urban planning, rapid urbanisation, crumbling infrastructure and inadequate drainage, the city proved yet again that it was woefully unprepared for the monsoon season.

With the rains comes a host of viral infections that seem to infiltrate water-logged cities around India every year. Nandita consulted a doctor who believed she had picked up a bug owing to the rains. The doctor gave her some medicines and sent her on her way.

But as weeks turned into months and the rains slowly retreated, her symptoms showed no sign of abating. The nausea, the vomiting, the pain, it became too much. Eventually, four months after being told she had a viral fever, she was diagnosed with tuberculosis (TB).

But it wasn't the most common type of TB that affects the lungs and causes persistent coughing, weight loss and loss of appetite that had infiltrated Nandita's body. Instead it was intestinal TB, a rare type of extra-pulmonary TB that is usually contracted by consuming uncooked meat or unpasturised milk. She was dumbfounded.

'I thought TB was something that only affected the lungs. How can bacteria enter my intestine out of nowhere? No one gave me any answers,' she says.

Nandita began an 18-month-long regime of swallowing 15 pills a day. The treatment worked but it came with side-effects like nausea and dizziness. The college life that Nandita had long dreamed of—one filled with late nights with new friends, inspiring conversations and extra-circular activities like dance—was overshadowed by this disease. Every day she approached her drugs with trepidation; the pills were so big that she felt like she would choke every time one went down her throat.

And as she was trying to cope with all the physical trauma that comes with contracting and treating TB, Nandita came up against another consequence of the disease, one that medicine couldn't treat.

'When I was diagnosed, the doctor told me in no uncertain terms: do not disclose your illness to anyone because it will impact your personal life in the future. She feared that I would be discriminated against,' she tells me, alluding to her marriage prospects.

Her fear was valid.

Eighteen months later, though, after swallowing hundreds of pills, Nandita was cured and she was able to finish her studies.

Not long afterwards Nandita moved to the capital, New Delhi, to embark on her post-graduate studies at the Indian Institute of Mass Communication. It was an opportunity for her to start afresh.

But not long after moving to New Delhi, that all too familiar lower abdominal pain came back. She dismissed it at first, recalling the promise that her doctor had made in Mumbai: that TB would never come back into her life. After all, she thought, it's probably the weather: New Delhi's heat by May is unbearable and causes all sorts of stomach aches and pains. The frequent power cuts across the city meant that cold goods like milk and paneer went sour quickly and so did the street food, lingering in the heat.

But as the pain persisted she knew something was wrong. On a hot May day, holding all her medical reports that her mother carried with her, the two sat in the doctor's clinic, clutching one another's hands. They were awaiting the results of Nandita's CT scan.

'Nandita, your TB has returned,' the doctor told her.

She was stunned.

Despite her diagnosis, the doctor assured Nandita that a small operation to remove the infected portion of her intestine would be enough to cure her. She could soon return to her normal life.

'My life came crashing down and I fell into pieces,' she says. 'The intensity of the bacteria was far more severe [this time], it was far more ravaging.'

But just when she thought things couldn't get any worse, they did.

✳

As old as known history, Mycobacterium tuberculosis, the bacteria that causes the disease, has plagued humankind for centuries. Spread through the air via coughing, spitting and speaking, it continues to claim more than one million lives every year.

In 1996, the World Health Organisation warned, 'In 1995, more people died of TB than in any other year in history. At least 30 million people will die from tuberculosis in the next ten years if current trends continue. Millions more will watch helplessly as friends and family members waste away, racked with coughing and sweating with fever. They may wish that medical science could cure this terrible disease.

The truth is, medical science can. Since 1952, the world has had effective and powerful drugs that could make every single TB patient well again' (World Health Organisation, 1996).

Fast-forward to 2017, which saw 10 million people contract the disease and 1.6 million die from it (World Health Organisation, 2018). The horrifying statistics make it not only the deadliest infectious disease in the world, but one of the world's top 10 killers globally, far ahead of HIV/AIDS.

But the world is letting people with TB down and nowhere else is that more evident than in India.

India accounts for the largest number of TB cases and deaths—it has 27 per cent of the global burden of cases and deaths (World Health Organisation, 2018). Ever year at least 400,000 people die of the disease and almost three million are infected (World Health Organisation, 2018). India also has the largest number of multiple-drug resistant TB cases (130,000)—patients who are resistant to at least two of the most powerful drugs used to cure the disease (World Health Organisation, 2018).

But the true burden of disease is unknown largely because of the private sector's failure to report confirmed cases to the government and the under-diagnosis of patients for reasons such as a lack of access to healthcare and poor diagnostic tests.

As we know, TB doesn't have to be a death sentence. As Mark Dybul, former executive director of the Global Fund to fight AIDS, Tuberculosis and Malaria, says: 'We have the tools to end TB as a pandemic and public health threat on the planet, but we are not doing it' (Koehring, 2014).

In the late 1940s effective drug treatments against TB became available and, in combination with economic and social development such as improved sanitary conditions and the development of food and trade surpluses, they enabled countries across western Europe and North America to significantly reduce their TB burden. But while the development of effective TB chemotherapy and modern-isation brought with it the expectation that TB would disappear in wealthier countries, the poor remained just as susceptible to the disease as ever before.

Nowadays, across Europe and the United States and as far as Australia, TB is no longer a public health threat.

'In short, the "forgotten plague" was forgotten in large part because it ceased to bother the wealthy,' Paul Farmer writes in *Infections and Inequalities* (Farmer, 2001, p.187).

Today, combating TB in poorer countries where poverty and social inequality is entrenched remains a distant hope. In India though, that distant hope is more like a futile dream, stoked by complacency, stigma and discrimination.

In the early 1990s India adopted DOTS (Directly Observed Treatment, Short Course)—a World Health Organisation-developed programme for ordinary TB infections. The strategy was specifically designed to ensure that all confirmed sputum smear positive patients (those who have tested positive on a microscopy TB test) would receive a standardised regimen of drugs for six to eight months, with at least the first two months being observed by a healthcare worker. While the strategy has changed over time to take into account the rise in drug-resistant cases and the increasing burden of TB and HIV co-infection, its goal has nevertheless remained the same: the provision of diagnosis, treatment and care for all patients.

But combating TB is not just about the provision of drugs—the socio-economic factors that drive the spread of the disease are just as critical as any medical intervention.

An inadequate healthcare system with too few diagnostic labora-tories, unaffordable medicines, drug stock-outs and a lack of trained staff combined with entrenched poverty has made India home to the world's largest epidemic of TB and drug-resistant TB.

The above coupled with overcrowded living conditions which enable the disease to spread rapidly, high rates of smoking and diabetes, air pollution, gender inequality, stigma, and poor nutrition has resulted in a public health crisis of epic proportions, a crisis so unrelenting that it kills one person every two minutes.

'We know most things about it, but TB still kills more people than any other pathogen, far more than alcoholism, AIDS, malaria, tropical diseases and Ebola combined, and nobody seems to care... Where is the shame? Where is the outrage?' (Reichman, 1997, p. 4).

*

Tuberculosis has always been associated with the notions of shame, guilt, isolation and rejection. Before the Industrial Revolution folklore often associated the disease with vampires (Tuberculosis and Vampire Myth, 2013). When one member of a family died from the disease and as other infected family members got progressively sick, people believed this was because the first person with TB drained the life from the others. By the nineteenth century, superstitions and beliefs around TB had evolved but fear remained ingrained in people's psyches. Colloquial names for the disease such as the 'white plague', with reference to the paleness common to those with TB, and 'consumption', reflecting the withering away of the infected body, had become commonplace (Tuberculosis and Vampire Myth, 2013). The disease eventually earned the nickname, 'Captain Among these Men of Death', before infections began to decline thanks to a greater understanding of the transmissibility of the disease along with a skin test, basic treatment and a vaccination (Rubin, 1995). The threat to European civilisation was over.

Stigma is an important social determinant of health. It is a process that begins when a particular trait or characteristic of an individual or group is identified as being undesirable or disvalued (Link and Phelan, cited in Courtwright and Turner, 2010). As a result, the stigmatised individual often internalises this sense of undesirability and adopts a set of attitudes about the characteristic including guilt, shame and disgust. Consequently, these attitudes produce a set of behaviours that include hiding the stigmatised trait, engaging in risky behaviour or withdrawing from relationships (Smith et al., cited in Courtwright and Turner, 2010).

Many academics argue that stigma could also be defined as a form of 'structural violence', a term coined by Norwegian sociologist Johan Galtung in the 1960s. Although the term conjures up images of physical violence, Galtung used the term to refer to social inequality—more specifically the social structures that cause harm by preventing people from accessing their basic needs such as education and healthcare. Galtung defines structural violence as an 'avoidable impairment of fundamental needs or, to put it in more general terms, the impairment of human life, which lowers the actual degree to which someone is able to meet their needs below that which would otherwise be possible' (Galtung, 1993).

Prominent medical anthropologist Dr Paul Farmer uses the term 'as a broad rubric that includes a host of offensives against human dignity; extreme and relative poverty, social inequalities ranging from racism to gender inequality, and the more spectacular forms of violence that are un-contestedly human rights abuses, some of them punishment for efforts to escape structural violence' (2004, p. 8).

But within the practice of medicine, in settings of great structural violence, doctors have not been trained to understand or alter social inequalities which become embodied as health disparities. 'Yet it has long been clear that many medical and public health interventions will fail if we are unable to understand the social determinants of disease' (Mosley and Chen, cited in Farmer et al., 2006).

Stigma can be defined as a form of 'structural violence' because it prevents people from accessing their basic needs such as healthcare. But research on stigma as a form of 'structural violence' is limited.

'As anthropologists, we see stigma research as frequently being too individualistically focused, and need to broaden the concept out to encompass historically determined and structural inequalities,' Ian Harper from the University of Edinburgh told the *Lancet* medical journal (Christodoulou, 2011).

In India, poverty is the root cause of TB. And the disease is shrouded in stigma because of its enduring association with marginalised and disenfranchised groups such as poor, low-caste slum dwellers.

TB thrives on people living in crowded living conditions, made worse by poor nutrition, HIV infection and a lack of access to healthcare. In India, a lack of knowledge about how TB is spread incites isolation, ostracisation, fear and rejection. Moreover, as the disease is perceived as a marker for HIV positivity, many people assume that someone who has TB must also be infected with HIV. Both diseases carry a deep fear of contagion and are linked to strong images of malnourished bodies and ultimately, death. Lastly, in India, TB stigma is also fuelled by superstition—the belief that the infected individual deserved it, that he or she has done something to warrant becoming infected.

'When people are stigmatised for having a particular disease there is usually an implicit assumption that they have brought it upon themselves and this helps justify the stigmatisation,' Anna Waldstien from the University of Kent also told the Lancet (Christodoulou, 2011).

'So, it becomes a socially constructed, self-fulfilling process.'

Of this stigma in India, it's women who are the worst affected.

✳

While the difficulties of treating TB are well-documented, there have been few attempts to understand the impact the disease can have on women.

Nevertheless, of the limited research that has been done, it has found that stigma around the disease is so strong that women who have TB or who are even suspected of having it have been abandoned by their families, shunned by their communities and harassed by healthcare workers. The same is not true for men. In environments where the disease is rampant, such as the slums of Mumbai, TB-related stigma is amplified, especially towards women whose social and economic foundations are shattered by it (Christodoulou, 2011).

A study on TB-related stigma among women in Kolkata, the capital of the eastern state of West Bengal, found that the widespread fear of contagion meant that communities took excessive precautions to be as far away from women as possible (Mukerji and Turan, 2018).

It didn't matter if they were a confirmed case or merely suspected of having TB, but women's families would do anything to avoid 'catching' the disease such as eating and sleeping separately and in doing so, stoke isolation and rejection.

But the discrimination even transcended physical boundaries.

'My nephew also told me, that if you talk to me on the phone then wipe the mouthpiece,' one woman told researchers from the University of Alabama (Mukerji and Turan, 2018, p. 730).

The study also found that women were victims of pervasive gossip and verbal abuse by their families and neighbours.

'When I walk they will say, "hey you, you stay away from us". It's not like I'm walking close to them. If they see me coming, they will go into their house … in case I stop, they say "that TB infected one is coming", they will go in saying, "she has come, she has come"… they say, "look she has come, the witch, the one who devours her own home, ever since this one has been born she has been devouring her home,"' a 20-year-old patient told researchers (Mukerji and Turan, 2018, p. 730).

Disease-related stigma can be so severe that women will go to extremes to delay diagnosis or keep their illness a secret for fear of being kicked out of their homes. In fact, every year it is estimated that 100,000 women suffering from TB are abandoned by their families, thrown out and left to fend for themselves because they are sick (Rao, 2015).

'How can it be that a disease that is somehow passable for a man can threaten the social fabric of a woman's life? What makes things worse is that they (women) depend on the very people who stigmatise them the most—their families and husbands—to take them to the doctor, to purchase medicines, to look after their children; and this dependence disables many women from fighting stigmatisation,' Dr Amrita Daftary, a TB researcher from McGill University in Canada, tells me.

'I think it is time we look at the root causes of stigma among women and these are inevitably social rather than individual. TB stigma in women is really a reflection of gender inequity.'

Not only are women discriminated against in their homes and rejected by their husbands, but unmarried women with TB are being taken off the 'marriage market' altogether. The study in Kolkata found that the loss of marital prospects was the most commonly reported concern among unmarried women (Mukerji and Turan, 2018). Some women reported that their engagements had been called off after the boy's family found out about the TB diagnosis. Other women feared that even after they were cured they wouldn't be able to get married and were scared they wouldn't be able to fulfil their duties as a wife and get pregnant.

'The thing is if boys have TB then people can ignore it. People are like yes, he had it, but he can get married ... but with girls it's like, she had it, so she can't. This is how our mindset is like,' a 20-year-old single woman told researchers (Mukerji and Turan, 2018, p. 731).

TB-related stigma can not only lead to significant delays in diagnosis but can also impact a woman's ability to complete her course of treatment.

Although noncompliance generally tops the list of favourite explanations why some women do not complete treatment, a woman's inability to complete her treatment is not a reflection of her unwillingness to nor is it a reflection of a lack of dedication to getting better. It's a by-product of the structural barriers that prevent women from accessing timely healthcare, and the failure of the healthcare system to take into account the impact of gender when providing care.

Women's health is undervalued and neglected so much so that society has conditioned women to believe their duty is to their family first and foremost and that their own health is inconsequential. As a result of being socially and economically dependent on their husbands, women's health is often ignored until the point where she can no longer perform her 'household duties'.

'When I cough then you guys never tell me to rest, but then you say "you have [a] disease you sit on one side",' one 45-year-old female patient told researchers (Mukerji and Turan, 2018, p. 731).

Even then though, when women are so obviously sick and require medical care, they are often forced to delay seeking care because they have duties to attend to and lack financial independence.

But the delay in seeking adequate healthcare only means that a woman stays infectious for longer, increasing the likelihood of her passing on the disease to her family. And so the vicious cycle of stigma continues.

When a woman does have contact with the public healthcare system, the way that TB is managed can reinforce the exclusion and isolation they already experience in their communities. For example, district tuberculosis officers in some parts of the country insist on verifying addresses before they dispense medicines. Given that women do not want everyone to know they have TB, they often give fake addresses or are put in a situation where they have no control over who in the community will know about their diagnosis. And as the treatment strategy for the disease—DOTS (Directly Observed Treatment, Short Course)—is community-based, the presence of TB nurses at someone's home, in addition to the location of DOTS clinics in communities, only fuels stigma. Because women's movements are closely monitored and gossiped about, a woman being spotted at a DOTS clinic can be so detrimental that she may decide to avoid treatment altogether for fear of being discovered by neighbours and family.

The structural barriers that impact a woman's ability to access healthcare such as a lack of autonomy, decision-making and control over earnings, coupled with the failure of the healthcare system to take into account the impact of gender on tuberculosis control, work hand-in-hand to worsen pre-existing gender-based health disparities.

✳

In July 2013, Nandita was wheeled into an operating theatre in Mumbai to remove part of her TB-infected intestine. She had hope though—after all, the doctor had assured her that a simple operation would mean that she could return to her studies in New Delhi soon. But a week after she was discharged from hospital, as she was recovering at her parents' home, she collapsed. She was rushed to hospital to find out that the operation on her abdomen hadn't in fact worked. In time she would have to have another five operations. She remained in hospital for three months, which turned into two years at home bed-ridden. Nandita was reduced to a mere skeleton at just 32 kilograms. Unable to eat, she survived on small sips of water for two months so the bacteria could be contained. But that wasn't the worst of it. What was worse than forgoing food for two months were the 96 injections of Kanamycin—a second-line drug for multiple-drug resistant TB (MDR-TB)—she had to endure on a daily basis. The oil-based injections were excruciating—so excruciating that it is not unusual for patients to refuse them and opt for death instead. When the nurse could no longer find veins in Nandita's hands for the injections, her neck was the next best option.

'With so many medications and intravenous fluids, I used to feel as if molten lava was running through my veins because it was that hot, it was that painful, and it was that raw. A foreigner had entered into my body and was eating away into my system slowly and steadily,' she says.

Within six months, Nandita had reached rock bottom.

Her fear of death was palpable. She went from a vivacious young woman with thick curly hair and a bright future to being reduced to a scrawny woman with all but a few strands of hair left on her head. She covered her fingers in superstitious rings—anything that could provide her with a glimmer of hope.

She thought life couldn't get worse. Then one day in late November 2013, she woke up from a nap and the room was silent. She could see her family talking, their lips and hands moving, but there was no sound. She thought she must still be dreaming. But no, she wasn't. Nandita had lost 90 per cent of her hearing—a side-effect of the Kanamycin injection.

The side-effects of Kanamycin are well-documented from hearing loss to renal failure. In fact, some studies suggest that one-third of MDR-TB patients who receive the injection lose their hearing (Linnert, 2015). Despite this, Nandita was never counselled by healthcare workers. She was never told that a single injection could mean that she would never hear even the simplest sounds like birds chirping on her balcony ever again.

'Kanamycin was the death. I was never told about it,' she says.

Nandita knew she would now face the double stigma of being a woman with TB and a disability. Her doctor had already told her not to disclose her TB diagnosis to anyone because it would harm her future marriage prospects. But now what would she tell people? That she woke up one day and she was suddenly deaf for no apparent reason? It devastated her.

She subsequently spiralled into a prolonged period of depression like so many other TB patients.

A World Health Organisation study found that one-third of female TB patients in the southern city of Chennai had psychosocial and emotional distress because of their diagnosis (2006). The distress of having the disease was often so extreme that it overshadowed the disease's physical symptoms. As one patient told researchers: 'I don't feel anything from my symptoms. Only the sadness, which makes me feel more dull' (World Health Organisation, 2006, p. 41). For some, the stigma, rejection and isolation was so bad that they had contemplated suicide. Other women reported that their husbands or in-laws wanted them to commit suicide.

✳

In 1986, India recorded its first case of human immunodeficiency virus (HIV), the virus that causes AIDS, among sex workers in the southern city of Chennai. The disease had only a few years previously garnered the public's attention in the United States after a few cases of rare diseases including Kaposi's sarcoma were reported among gay men in New York and California. But it was six years after India had confirmed cases of HIV that the government responded. After all, HIV wasn't a priority with only 96 AIDS cases and 5879 people infected with the virus (Rao, 2017, p. 202). But a few things made the government feel compelled to act: widespread media reports of discrimination of HIV patients, denial of treatment by healthcare workers, suicides driven by stigma, shame and rejection, and abandonment of dead bodies, with no one willing to cremate them (Rao, 2017, p.202).

In 1992, India created its National AIDS Control Programme (NACP), implemented by the National AIDS Control Organisation (NACO) under the Ministry of Health and Family Welfare. In its initial stages the programme was focused on understanding the burden of HIV and epidemiological trends. It has since evolved into a major HIV prevention and treatment programme.

Since 1986, the HIV epidemic in India has mushroomed to an estimated 2.1 million people living with the virus, as of 2016 (UNAIDS, n.d.). Every year, approximately 80,000 people are newly infected and an estimated 69,000 die of AIDS-related diseases such as tuberculosis (UNAIDS, n.d.).

In 2004, free HIV treatment—antiretroviral therapy (ART)—became available. Today it is estimated that 49 per cent of HIV-infected people across the country are on life-saving treatment (UNAIDS, n.d.).

Despite having the third-largest epidemic in the world after South Africa and Nigeria, (which is a result of its huge population) India is part of the global success story in being able to reduce infections and increase free access to life-saving ART. Since 2010, new HIV infections in India have decreased by 56 per cent and AIDS-related deaths have decreased by 22 per cent (UNAIDS, n.d.). It is incredible progress against a disease that was not long ago considered a death sentence.

But this is not the whole story.

The HIV epidemic has historically been entwined with fear of contagion, with disturbing images of malnourished, rash-ridden bodies and death. It has also been associated with the question of sexual mortality and with marginalised groups who are, in many parts of the world, considered to be immoral such as men who have sex with men.

Statistics show that men who have sex with men are 28 times more likely to be infected with HIV than the general population because of biological, behavioural and legal factors which place them at higher risk of infection (UNAIDS, 2018, p.14). However, despite this, HIV disproportionately affects adolescent girls and women because of their unequal status in society. In India, 'the impact of HIV/AIDS for most men', a UNAIDS report writes, has been 'cushioned by their privileged position in society' (Bharat, Aggleton and Tyrer, 2001, p.42). For women, meanwhile, it has 'intensified' (Bharat, Aggleton and Tyrer, 2001, p.42). While there are biological factors which make women more prone to infection than men during heterosexual sex— such as the fact that women have a larger mucosal surface exposed during sex—there are socio-cultural reasons why some women face increased vulnerability to infection.

For one, women often have little power or control over the sexual behaviour of their partners, such as the ability to negotiate condom use or to say no. Many Indian women are also vulnerable to coerced sex including marital rape which makes it difficult to protect themselves for fear of violence. Despite repeated calls by female activists and women themselves to make marital rape a crime, it has fallen on deaf ears. In fact, Narendra Modi's government recently said that criminal-ising marital rape would 'destabilise the institution of marriage' and could become an easy tool to 'harass husbands' (Choudhury, 2018). Such attitudes towards women make it difficult for them to protect themselves against HIV, gender-based violence and intimate partner violence. As one young HIV-positive Indian woman told researchers: 'My husband had AIDS explained to him but he had sex with me that same night. I asked him if it was OK but he said there was no problem. Under the influence of alcohol, he doesn't listen to me. What could I do?' (Bharat, Aggleton and Tyrer, 2001, p.43).

These factors, combined with a lack of access to healthcare and education; poverty which can mean that adolescent girls and women are propelled into partaking in transactional sex or early or forced marriage; and gender inequality, place women and girls at a heightened risk of contracting HIV.

Consequently, while India has made tremendous progress in reducing the number of new infections every year and getting more and more people on treatment, the reality is that HIV stigma, influenced by gender inequality and social norms, has led to a disproportionate death rate for women (Rathis, cited in Avert, 2019).

✳

In 1999, Mona Balani's husband tested positive for HIV. Not long after, Mona also tested positive.

She was 24 years old at the time; the couple had a newborn and a toddler and were living in Jaipur, the capital of the western Indian state of Rajasthan.

Mona had heard about HIV in tenth grade at school. But she just knew HIV to be AIDS, which equated to death. 'It was like there was a death warrant out for us,' she says about finding out she and her husband were positive.

Instead of counting on her in-laws' support, she was blamed; they believed it was Mona's fault her husband had contracted HIV. Mona stood there as her husband's family told him: 'Due to Mona you got HIV. Why? Because she is educated. She went to college. Maybe she had some boyfriends and maybe she had multiple relationships. Due to her you got HIV.'

One year after their diagnosis, Mona's husband contracted TB. At first it was regular TB—the type that affects the lungs—which can be cured within six to eight months. But it spread, first to his spine, then to his knees, brain and eyes. Five years later he lost his battle against the disease that had ravaged his body. It was the second death in Mona's family within three years—in 2002 their two-and-a-half-year-old son lost his 13-month-long battle with TB. Their son was never tested for HIV.

In addition to caring for her husband and son and battling her own HIV infection, Mona had also suffered TB of the lungs. But her health wasn't a priority.

'The status of women is sub-standard,' Mona tells me at her office in New Delhi where she works at the India HIV/AIDS Alliance, a non-profit organisation that supports community action to prevent HIV infection.

'Being a woman my priority is my family, not me. First I have to feed my husband, then I have to feed my children. Even though I am hungry, even though I am sick, it doesn't matter.'

And then in 2006, Mona's TB came back.

Her weight plummeted from 65 kilograms to a mere 30 kilograms. She was skeletal, so thin that her eyes had sunken into the back of her head. The few work prospects she had dried up—no one would hire her because she looked too frail. But doctor after doctor ignored her symptoms. It took her a year and a half before she was able to get a diagnosis: she had intestinal TB—the same type that Nandita had.

When she began treatment she simultaneously began ART for her HIV infection, which had since become available in the public health sector for free. But the medicines led to side-effects such as skin rashes and boils—side-effects that were nor overly disturbing or concerning, but rather common. When she went to a local government hospital in search of a nurse to dress the boil that was weeping on her foot, she was denied treatment. As the nurse began dressing Mona's wound with naked hands, Mona interrupted and told the nurse, 'Please stop, I am living with HIV, you have to wear gloves'. The nurse screamed, 'HIV! You have to go to a district hospital.' She continued to yell and point saying, 'Doctor, she is an AIDS person.'

But even as time went on and India scaled up free HIV treatment across the country, which meant that patients have undetectable virus loads and therefore are unable to transmit the virus, Mona has continued to face stigma.

Not long ago she went to a private dentist for a check-up in New Delhi. As the dentist was about to open her mouth she requested he put on gloves. 'Doctor please put on gloves because I have HIV,' she told him. 'You have HIV? You have to go. You have to go to a different dental hospital,' he replied. He placed his sickle probe down and walked out of the room. Mona lay in the dental chair, no longer dumbfounded by the stigma she continues to face to this day, stigma she knows is inordinate because she is a woman.

'I am always ashamed to tell people I'm living with HIV. I'm afraid to be open about my status,' she tells me. 'Every step there is fear with me, that I should not talk, that I should not eat with someone because I have HIV, that I should not shake hands with someone because I have HIV.'

'Stigma is all around. Most of the time it [leads to] delay in diagnosis and treatment.'

✳

Stigma associated with HIV has long been recognised as a major barrier in the fight against the disease. It is a major barrier in the uptake of testing and treatment. The disease, like TB, is considered a disease of 'others'—of those living on the margins of society. Fear of contagion and a lack of awareness about how HIV spreads only works to deepen this stigma. Unlike TB, which is strongly linked to poverty, HIV is equated with promiscuity and sexual deviance; with people whose social and sexual behaviour doesn't fit the mold of what is considered acceptable. But in India, stigma is also fuelled by gender inequality. Stigma itself is a gendered phenomenon which continues to threaten the country's ability to combat its epidemic.

A groundbreaking study into HIV stigma and discrimination in India revealed huge disparities in the treatment of women and men who had the disease (Bharat, Aggleton and Tyrer, 2001). The study, carried out in Mumbai and Bengaluru, the capital of the southern state of Karnataka, found that HIV-positive women were characterised as being of 'loose character' and blamed by their in-laws for infecting their sons—just like Mona. 'My mother-in-law tells everybody, "because of her, my son got this disease. My son is a simple boy as good as gold—but she brought him this disease",' an HIV-positive 26-year-old woman told researchers (Bharat, Aggleton and Tyrer, 2001, p.41).

Even when parents knew their son had visited sex workers, they had the audacity to blame the wife because she failed in her duty to keep her husband 'under control'. When sons died from the disease, in most cases the daughter-in-law was thrown out of the house and left to fend for herself and her family. As one HIV-positive woman who was thrown out after her husband died said: 'My in-laws have said, "Now we have no use of you in our home". I wish I could die, then I won't have to think where to go' (Bharat, Aggleton and Tyrer, 2001, p.45). Whereas women are seen as harbingers of disease, unable to control their husbands' sexual urges, men are seen as incapable of doing wrong, cushioned by their privilege in a patriarchal society.

But stigma is not only confined to the home, it extends to healthcare workers too—the very people who are meant to provide treatment and support. A recent study in Mumbai and Bengaluru found that up to 80 per cent of healthcare workers in government and private clinics were willing to prohibit women living with HIV from having children, and that up to 83 per cent of respondents felt that women who acquired HIV through sex or drugs 'got what they deserved' (Ekstrand et al., 2013). Research also found that pregnant HIV-positive women were repeatedly refused healthcare and delivery services and that some pregnant women were told to get an abortion (Bharat, Aggleton and Tyrer, 2001, p.43). Moreover, the narratives revealed that stigma even extended to women who accompanied their HIV-positive husbands to hospital for healthcare. As one woman told researchers: 'In the hospital the staff used to say, "Why are you coming to the hospital. Didn't you know when you first made the mistake?" I used to feel so embarrassed and also angry with my husband. But what's the use of getting angry now?' (Bharat, Aggleton and Tyrer, 2001, p.43). A study examining the impact stigma can have on HIV-positive rural women found that over 70 per cent had been physically threatened by healthcare workers and two-thirds had been denied medical care (Nyamathi et al., 2011).

It is no surprise that stigma can have a devastating impact on a woman's ability to access HIV testing and treatment. It is no surprise that women, fearing stigma, are less likely to access testing, and those who do know they are HIV-positive are less likely to disclose their status (Nyamathi et al., 2013).

✳

When Deepti Chavan contracted tuberculosis again at the age of 16, she knew the drill: six to eight months of pills and then she would be cured. She thought she knew what fighting the disease would require because she'd already been through it at the age of 11. Growing up in India's TB capital, Mumbai, she'd contracted the disease as a child, she believes, from travelling on overcrowded local trains to and from school. But the TB that ravaged her body for the second time was not as simple as taking pills for six months.

Just as she was preparing for her board examinations to complete high school, she began to feel sick. It was the cough. It was like someone had taken a razor blade to her throat. It wouldn't stop. She went to a doctor who prescribed medicine for it and sent Deepti on her way. But the cough persisted. Eventually the doctor suggested she get an x-ray. It took about a month, but finally Deepti was diagnosed— her TB had come back. So she began a daily routine of medicines feeling optimistic that within six months or so she would be cured. But unlike last time, the pills didn't help. Her health continued to deteriorate—weight loss, fever, night sweats became all too common. Her parents took her to a chest physician who they hoped could help. He chopped and changed her drugs. But the new pills didn't work and Deepti continued her downward spiral.

A few months later Deepti's doctor told her she had a dangerous type of TB—multiple-drug resistant TB (MDR-TB). The drugs she had been swallowing for the past several months had been of no use because she was resistant to them. The doctor, working in the MDRT-TB capital of the world, didn't know because he hadn't ordered a drug susceptibility test which would have determined which TB drugs Deepti would be sensitive to and if she had drug-resistance. She was told she would have to undergo an operation to remove the infected part of her lung.

'I just knew that TB was meant to be this disease that gets cured within six to eight months of treatment. I didn't know what MDR-TB meant. No one explained anything,' she says.

As Deepti underwent an operation on her lung, the surgeon found that both the upper and lower lobe of it was infected with deadly bacteria. Because of her age and vulnerability he couldn't remove it all.

So she continued taking up to 20 pills a day along with the dreaded Kanamycin injection. The side-effects were excruciating: coughing up blood, blurry vision, hearing problems and severe joint pain that made it difficult to get out of bed. 'I stopped looking in the mirror as I was scared of what I would see,' she says.

But her health continued to deteriorate. Her plan of attending university to study engineering looked increasingly dubious. Doctors told Deepti and her family that she had six months to live. They said there was nothing they could do.

'Doctors said, "just take the medicines" but they were unsure whether they would help. They told me that I would eventually die, that in six months I will die. They told my parents to stop wasting their time on me,' she says.

Her family sold everything they could to find a surgeon who would be willing to operate on Deepti. Surgeon after surgeon told Deepti she had six months to live and a one per cent chance of survival if she was operated on. When a surgeon finally agreed, Deepti thought: If I'm going to die any way, why not fight one last time?

She went into the operation singing her favourite song. Whatever the outcome, the surgery would end her suffering. If it were a success, she would survive. If it weren't, she would die and be finally put out of her misery.

Against all odds, she survived.

'Doctors kept telling me the same thing: that I was going to die. Everyone thought I wouldn't make it. That's the mistake they made. You cannot tell someone they're going to die. If they're going to die, then they're going to die. No one can prepare you for death. What if I had given up? What if my parents had stopped everything and let me die?'

As Deepti recovered in hospital and relatives came to visit, the most pertinent question wasn't: How are you feeling? Instead it was: who will marry you now that you have lost a lung? Deepti was dumbfounded. She had, in spite of everything, just survived a highly risky operation. She still had a long way to go to recover from the disease, but she had survived. Wasn't that cause for celebration?

'I was taken aback because I had just gotten out of a major surgery that was life-threatening and people were only interested in who will marry me. Everyone told me that no one should know I had TB, that I shouldn't tell anyone … because no one will marry me,' she says.

Six years after her diagnosis, six years of taking thousands of drugs, 400 Kanamycin injections and two major lung operations, in 2005 Deepti was cured. But while she was cured of a disease that had devastated her body, she still wasn't well: she had to undergo several stomach operations because of the damage all the drugs had done.

'Nothing is normal. Even once you're cured, your life isn't the same afterwards.'

Society had conditioned Deepti to believe that she was unworthy of marriage, that because she'd had a disease that was associated with poverty and she had lost a lung, no one would love her.

But she found love online in 2004 and married in 2011. She was shocked that despite telling her husband about her illness, he wanted to marry her. Her first instinct was to say no.

'I didn't think that he deserved to marry someone like me.'

Both Deepti and Nandita hope that speaking out about their experiences as women they can help dispel myths and fight stigma.

'People assume that if a woman is infected with TB she might not be able to conceive. People also think that an ill woman is less competent to look after the family,' Deepti says. 'We need to emphasise that TB can happen to anyone, [and] it's a treatable and curable disease.'

Both women are members of Survivors Against TB, a community-based movement led by survivors who are working to strengthen India's fight against the disease. The group wants to highlight that in patriarchal society women who have TB not only have to live with the disease on a daily basis, but they have to fight gender-based stigma and structural barriers that hamper their ability to access diagnosis and treatment. They want to highlight the fact that TB kills more women in India than maternal deaths every year and yet despite the shocking figures, the TB epidemic is not viewed as a gendered one. The group wants gender-specific sensitisation programmes to educate women to give them the confidence to seek treatment and it wants the healthcare system to stop abandoning women. It wants policy-makers and healthcare workers to think about alternative methods of providing TB treatment, to think about gender appropriate TB interventions that make it easier for women to access and remain on treatment.

Nandita is also fighting to ensure that newer drugs that are safer and more effective are made affordable and accessible to everybody with drug-resistant TB. She does not want anyone else to go through daily injections of toxic drugs that can lead to hearing loss. She, and another female TB survivor, has filed a patent challenge to prevent the pharmaceutical company Johnson & Johnson (J&J) from extending its monopoly on the TB drug bedaquiline—a drug that is recommended by the WHO for MDR-TB but few have access to because of its high price.

✳

It's a sticky summer morning in New Delhi. It's early but already the heat and haze is overwhelming. I'm on my way to hear Nandita speak at a conference. For almost two years we've been talking through Google chat but we have never met. We look for one another in the conference room, and when we find one another we embrace like old friends. We rely on text messages, hand-written notes and slow, articulate speech to converse because of Nandita's hearing loss.

She takes to the stage to tell her story, a story so heart-rending and heart-felt that everyone in the audience stands up to applaud, many with tears in their eyes.

'If you think I'm going to keep quiet today, let me tell you that is not the case. It has reached a breaking point now that people are frustrated with the pain they're suffering. It is only when we all come together collectively that we can defeat this disease,' she tells the audience.

Her words reverberate around the room. Everyone nods their heads. Nandita is on a mission and no one is getting in her way. Female TB survivors are fighting back.

References

Avert (2019) *HIV and AIDS in India*. Available at: https://www.avert.org/professionals/hiv-around-world/asia-pacific/india#footnote84_p5fq9g9

Bharat, S., Aggleton, P. and Tyrer, P. (2001) *India: HIV and AIDS-related Discrimination, Stigmatization and Denial*. UNAIDS. Available at: http://data.unaids.org/publications/irc-pub02/jc587-india_en.pdf

Christodoulou, M. (2011) The stigma of tuberculosis. *The Lancet* 11(9): 663–664. Available at: https://www.download.thelancet.com/journals/laninf/article/PIIS1473-3099(11)70228-6/fulltext

Choudhury, S. (2018) Why is outlawing marital rape still a distant dream in India?, *The Wire*, 28 October. Available at: https://thewire.in/law/india-marital-rape-criminal-law

Courtwright, A. and Turner, A. N. (2010) Tuberculosis and stigmatization: Pathways and interventions. *Public Health Reports* 125 (Suppl 4): 34–42. Available at: https://journals.sagepub.com/doi/10.1177/00333549101250S407

Ekstrand, M. L., Ramakrishna, J., Bharat, S. et al. (2013) Prevalence and drivers of HIV stigma among health providers in urban India: implications for interventions. *Journal of the International AIDS Society* 16 (3Suppl2): 18717. Available at: https://onlinelibrary.wiley.com/doi/full/10.7448/IAS.16.3.18717

Farmer, P. (2001) *Infections and Inequalities: The Modern Plagues*. California: University of California Press.

Farmer, P. (2004) *Pathologies of Power: Health, Human Rights, and the New War on the Poor*. California: University of California Press.

Farmer, P. E., Nizeye, B., Stulac, S. et al. (2006) Structural violence and clinical medicine. *Radiologic Clinics of North America* 33(4): 619–39.

Galtung, J. (1993) 'Kulturelle Gewalt', *Der Burger im Staat 1993*; 43:106–12.

Koehring, M. (2014) Ancient enemy, modern imperative. *The Economist*, June 30. Available at: https://eiuperspectives.economist.com/healthcare/ancient-enemy-modern-imperative

Linnert, M. (2015) Almost deaf due to meds—but there is hope. *TB Proof*, 8 July. Available at: http://www.tbproof.org/deaf-due-meds-hope/

Mukerji, R. and Turan, J. M. (2018) Exploring manifestations of TB-related stigma experienced by women in Kolkata, India. *Annals of Global Health*

84(*4*): 727–735. Available at: https://www.annalsofglobalhealth.org/articles/10.29024/aogh.2383/

Nyamathi, A. M., Sinha, S., Ganguly, K. et al. (2011) Challenges experienced by rural women in India living with AIDS and implications for the delivery of HIV/AIDS Care. *Health Care for Women International* 32(—): 300–313. Available at: https://www.tandfonline.com/doi/abs/10.1080/07399332.2010.536282

Nyamathi, A. M., Ekstrand, M., Gilburne, J. Z. et al. (2013) Correlates of stigma among rural Indian women living with HIV/AIDS. *AIDS and Behavior* 17(*1*): 329–339. Available at: https://link.springer.com/article/10.1007%2Fs10461-011-0041-9

Rao, M. (2015) The gendered delay in the diagnosis and treatment of tuberculosis patients in India. *The Caravan*, 23 September. Available at: https://caravanmagazine.in/vantage/gendered-delay-diagnosing-tuberculosis-patients

Rao, S. (2017) *Do We Care: India's Health System*. India: Oxford University Press.

Reichman, L. B. (1997) Tuberculosis Elimination- What's to stop us? (counterpoint). *The International Journal of Tuberculosis and Lung Disease* 1(*1*): 3–11.

Rubin, S. A. (1995) Tuberculosis: Captain of all these men of death. *Radiologic Clinics of North America* 33(*4*):619–39.

Tuberculosis and the Vampire Myth (2013) *Aeras*, 30 October. Available at: http://www.aeras.org/blog/tuberculosis-and-the-vampire-myth#.XJEEXygza01

UNAIDS n.d., 'Country- India'. United Nations. Available at: http://www.unaids.org/en/regionscountries/countries/india

UNAIDS (2018) *Miles to Go: Closing Gaps, Breaking Barriers, Righting Injustices*. United Nations. Available at: http://www.unaids.org/sites/default/files/media_asset/miles-to-go_en.pdf

World Health Organisation (1996) Groups at risk: WHO report on the tuberculosis epidemic 1996. United Nations. Available at: https://www.who.int/tb/publications/groups-risk-report/en/

World Health Organisation (2018) *Global Tuberculosis Report 2018*. United Nations. Available at: https://www.who.int/tb/publications/global_report/en/

World Health Organisation (2006) Gender and tuberculosis: Cross-site analysis and implications of a multi-country study in Bangladesh, India, Malawi, and Colombia. United Nations. Available at: https://www.who.int/tdr/publications/documents/sebrep3.pdf

CHAPTER 6

Invisible Women*
Injecting Drug Users

It's late May in Imphal, the capital of the north-eastern Indian state of Manipur. The rains haven't arrived yet despite heavy clouds hanging in the crevasses of the rich green mountains which surround the city. The cool air is a welcome reprieve from the stifling heat of New Delhi and the sticky humidity of Mumbai. At most state capital airports, you land on the tarmac, pick up your luggage and simply walk through the exit. But Imphal is different. As a foreigner I'm escorted to a desk where I show my passport and answer a series of questions. What are you doing in Manipur? Why would you come here? How long will you be here for? Who is your guide? As a foreigner you need a guide to enter the state—someone who, at the very least, will tell the authorities that he or she is responsible for you during your stay. I'd arranged for a young university student to be my sponsor in advance and the authorities wasted no time in calling her, and the hotel I said I was staying at, to check that this was true.

---

* Parts of this chapter has been published previously as Sophie Cousins, Invisible women: The unseen plight of Manipur's female drug users, *The Caravan*, 1 September 2017. Available at: https://caravanmagazine.in/reportage/unseen-plight-manipur-female-drug-users

Despite being a small city, the streets of Imphal are chaotic, filled with old rickshaws, decaying taxis and trucks spewing black fumes. They are also filled with armed security forces. A lot of the roads are unpaved and deeply pot-holed and as traffic drives by, they collect the dust and send it like balloons into the air.

The dust, dirt and fumes stick to your face, get under your fingernails and filter deep into your lungs. It's easy to see why so many people wear face masks: the lack of paved roads, coupled with the abundance of old vehicles and burning of rubbish on the side of the road, has created conditions reminiscent of Kathmandu, one of the most polluted cities in the world.

In the centre of Imphal is the Mothers' Market, otherwise known as Ima Keithel, a sprawling food and goods market run entirely by women. It's the epicentre, the heart of an otherwise nondescript, uninspiring city. There are few cafes and no bars—alcohol is banned in Manipur. Unlike the bustling capital cities of other states where local and international chains have popped up for the urbanised, affluent youth, there is no Café Coffee Day, certainly no Starbucks and nothing like a Subway in sight. Pork and fish are the staples here, along with steaming momos—dumplings that are cooked in oversized pots along the side-streets.

At Ima Keithel, thousands of women sell everything from fresh fish to jewellery from dawn to dusk every day. It has become so popular, perhaps for a lack of other income-generating opportunities, that stalls have sprawled out beyond the confines of the market. Hundreds of women have set up shop outside its entrance on the sidewalks. Ima Keithel is poetic and rhythmic and representative of the prominent position women have historically played in Manipuri society. Centuries ago when Manipuri men were off fighting wars with the Chinese and Burmese, it was the women who were left at home, responsible for looking after their families. The market embodies women's strength and resilience, even today.

✳

On the outskirts of Imphal, nestled amid the rice paddies, is an abandoned red-brick house. Overgrown grass and weeds surround the house which has no front door, only a chain with a bolted padlock. Rubbish is strewn across the front lawn, including old pairs of children's shoes. Perhaps a family used to live here, I wonder, or perhaps children live here now. A girl, no older than seven, runs to the front of the house and unlocks the chained gate. She struggles for a minute, it's heavy in her hands, before one of the men waiting outside helps her. Inside the house appears as if it's still being constructed—piles of wood and other building materials are piled up on the concrete floors.

Mud-ridden footprints on the ground lead to a back room where people and used needles litter the floor. Bed sheets hang across the two wide windows in the left corner of the room. They're not big enough though and a few beams of glaring sunlight shine through the otherwise pitch dark room. There are about 10 people, some women, some men. A few are sprawled out on mattresses that adorn the otherwise sparse room while others kneel next to a timber table which has drugs and needles spread across it. Some appear dishevelled and lost; others are dressed in work attire, like they've stepped out on their lunch break for a hit. The group have gathered to inject heroin and inhale WY—a bright red tablet of methamphetamine and caffeine which translates literally to mean 'mad drug'.

A young barefoot girl—the same girl who unlocked the chain at the front of the house—stands in the corner of the room like a headmistress minding her students. When people need water to clean their needles or to swish around their mouth they throw up their hands. She immediately runs and gets some from the tap. They don't seem to mind its salient feature: its murky, light brown colour.

It's here where Jenny, a 46-year-old former school teacher, comes to get her daily dose. She's homeless and buys drugs here every day to later sell on the streets to survive. She sells sex too.

Jenny has a sunken face and greying hair that she ties in a low bun behind her ears. She dresses in traditional Manipuri clothes, donning a long dark green patterned skirt and a white shirt. As a former school teacher, her command of the English language is superb and her love of the language is evident. She is proud of the career she had and talks about it with enthusiasm and a hint of nostalgia.

Jenny and I crowd around the small timber table as Imphal's head drug dealer—a middle-aged woman who doesn't want to talk—gets out the white powder. She divides it into small piles before filling baggies with it. Each bag is ₹100 (US$1.40) worth of heroin—enough for one shot. Jenny buys a few bags and safely puts them in the inner zipper of her purse.

'At first I couldn't stand [heroin]—it was very hard. But the next time I felt like chasing it. It's very good at getting rid of all the problems in my life,' she tells me.

Jenny places a WY tablet on a strip of aluminum foil, heats it from below with a lighter and breathes in the fumes, exhaling huge clouds of smoke. She then gets out a needle and a syringe and fills it with heroin.

'I'm sorry you have to see this. Don't ever do drugs,' she says.

＊

The National Aids Control Organisation (NACO) estimates there are 200,000 injecting drug users in India (NACO, n.d.). Other research puts the figure significantly higher at up to 1.1 million drug users across the country (Aceijas et al., 2006). Most users are concentrated in the north-east of the country—primarily in Manipur and Nagaland—but are growing in northern states including Punjab. Prime Minister Narendra Modi has described drug addiction as a 'menace' synonymous with three D's: 'darkness, destruction, and devastation' ('Modi's Mann ki Baat', 2014).

The most commonly injected substances in India are heroin and opioid pharmaceuticals such as Spasmo-Proxyvon (Armstrong et al., 2014). The typical drug user in India is male, aged between 15 and 35, uneducated and unemployed (Medhi et al., 2011). However, up to 20 per cent of drug users are female (Wherley and Chatterjee, 2015). Despite making up an estimated one-fifth of injecting drug users, there is a paucity of research on this group of women who, as a result, remain misunderstood and largely invisible, their voices seldom heard.

Numerous factors have led to widespread drug use in north-east India. For one, the states of Manipur, Mizoram and Nagaland share a long, porous border with Myanmar, the world's second-largest producer of opium, after Afghanistan. The similar is true of Punjab in northern India which shares a border with Pakistan, which borders Afghanistan, making it a major transit route in the international drug smuggling trade.

In addition to its proximity to Myanmar, both Nagaland and Manipur are characterised by long-standing civil insurgency. For decades dozens of different armed groups have been fighting to either secede from those states, or from India as a whole. The north-east is geographically isolated from mainland India—it is separated by Bangladesh—and many people belong to indigenous tribes that are ethnically, linguistically and culturally distinct from one another and especially from the rest of India (Kermode et al., 2010).

The ongoing conflicts have had a profound impact on the communities in the north-east. According to Human Rights Watch, it has led to 'decades of neglect, widespread corruption, and a failure by successive governments to deliver economic growth and sustainable development' (2008). The civil insurgent movements have also led to a large Indian military presence and the implementation of the Armed Forces (Special Powers) Act of 1958 which grants security forces broad powers to use legal force and provides near immunity from prosecution.

A major consequence of decades of neglect and stunted economic growth is that Manipur is also plagued by a widespread job shortage—as of 2016, almost 750,000 of the state's 2.7 million residents were unemployed (Cousins, 2017).

High unemployment, coupled with geographical isolation, the easy availability of drugs, lack of development, and the local socio-cultural and political context are big drivers of drug use among men. With a rich tribal history, masculinity in the north-east is 'influenced by a convergence of the traditional/tribal male warrior role' which bonds young people together through social networks based on neighbourhood and tribal groupings (McDuie-Ra, 2012 cited in Armstrong et al., 2014).

Research shows that initiation into injecting drug use in Manipur among men is a common social activity and therefore to some extent is normalised (Kermode, 2007).

Consequently, injecting drug use has become a rite of passage among the masses—an opportunity for young men to bond with friends and prove their masculinity. Male injecting drug users in the north-east, however, differ from those in other parts of the country in that they are more likely to be young, well educated and living with their families (Kermode, 2007).

But the reasons why men and women fall into drug use differ starkly.

'My anecdotal impression is that guys are more likely to get into drug use because of boredom and wanting to have some fun, but become addicted over time,' a global health expert who has extensively researched female injecting drug users in Manipur tells me.

'Whereas women tend to drift into drug use because they are socio-economically vulnerable and the drugs help them to deal with their pain.'

Women, the expert tells me, 'often enter drug use with a history of losing their family or dysfunctional family relationships, and even if they had family before drug use, they've very unlikely to have an ongoing relationship with them now.'

Her anecdotal insight (she wants to remain anonymous for fear of jeopardising her work) is supported by research that has found many female drug injecting users were living in vulnerable circumstances at the time of drug initiation and were introduced to injecting without completely understanding what it involved and its consequences (Kermode et al., 2009).

'I had run away from home. My parents died, so we were looked after by our aunty at her place. One day I ran away from home and ended up in the railway station. There I met these new friends.

They told me that if I injected the white substance I would feel better—I would be able to forget all my sorrows. So I injected for the first time,' an 18-year-old drug user told researchers (Kermode et al., 2009).

In fact, a recent study by the United Nations Office on Drugs and Crime (UNODC) found that Manipur has the highest ratio of female to male users in all north-eastern states—28.2 per cent of injecting users in the state are women (Kumar et al., 2015, p. 15). The study also found that more than one-fourth of female injecting drug users were widowed or separated and that one-third of women sold drugs or sex to survive, just like Jenny does.

So while drug use is considered a rite of passage for young men, women instead are propelled into a vicious cycle of drug use and drug selling, violence and sex work. And in doing so, they face serious threats to their health, safety and well-being. They face gender-based violence, human rights violations, high rates of incarceration and stigma and discrimination. But despite the figures that illustrate that women make up a significant proportion of drug users—particularly in the north-east—they are rarely found in research, harm reduction programmes or the healthcare system. They are an invisible, hidden, silent population.

*

Opiate substitution therapy (OST) is a way of treating opiate addiction by supplying illegal drug users, such as heroin users, with medically prescribed drugs such as methadone or buprenorphine. These legal alternatives, which are usually given in tablet or liquid form in a clinical setting, are longer-acting than their illegal cousins, but produce less of a high. This helps reduce the user's cravings and withdrawal symptoms.

The effectiveness of OST has led it to become the first-line treatment for opioid addiction and a critical element in the prevention of HIV infection among injecting drug users. Not only has OST emerged as a frontline treatment, but opiate dependence is now recognised as a chronic relapsing condition similar to other non-communicable diseases such as diabetes. Viewing drug addiction as a health issue—for which users need accessible, long-lasting treatment—has helped to increase OST's acceptability in some parts of the world and has, as a result, increased access to it.

Research illustrates wide-ranging benefits of OST, including reduced drug use, reduced risk of contracting HIV and other blood-borne diseases, reduced criminal behaviour, and reduced deaths from overdoses (Kermode et al., 2011). Importantly, OST provides a critical opportunity to connect drug users with the healthcare system—people who would otherwise likely have little or no contact with it.

In doing so it enables the provision of a broader harm reduction strategy which includes access to clean needles and syringes, primary medical care and other services such as HIV testing and antiretroviral therapy, and testing and treatment for other infectious diseases such as tuberculosis and hepatitis C.

But while there are an estimated 11.8 million people who inject drugs worldwide, only eight per cent have access to OST (Kermode et al., 2011). Global inequity is stark. For example, 90 per cent of injecting drug users in the United Kingdom are receiving OST; in India, that figure stands at three per cent (Kermode et al., 2011).

On paper though, India has embraced OST.

The country licensed buprenorphine for the treatment of opioid dependence in drug treatment centres in 1999. In 2008, OST was incorporated into the National AIDS Control Programme's (NACO) harm reduction efforts (Rao et al., 2014). OST was initially available at licensed non-governmental organisations (NGOs) and delivered through drop-in-centres but in 2010 it was expanded to government hospitals. Then, in 2012, India was hailed for its introduction of the country's first methadone maintenance treatment centre. Methadone is a more powerful opiate than buprenorphine for users with more serious addiction.

But while India has theoretically embraced OST, the reality on the ground paints a very different picture, especially for female injecting drug users.

❊

The National AIDS Control Organisation (NACO) has clinical practice guidelines for treating opioid addiction with OST which specify particular considerations for female injecting drug users. Recognising that females face far-reaching challenges in accessing OST, the guidelines stipulate that: special efforts must be made to make the female injecting drug user comfortable as females are often reluctant to access services at places with predominantly male clients; a doctor and counsellor must ensure that the female is examined and interviewed in the presence of female staff; during the assessment, enquiries must be made about the symptoms of sexually transmitted infections, last menstrual period and child-bearing history; females must be given priority during follow-up and dispensing of OST medicines and not be made to wait their turn; contraception must be offered to women in their child-bearing period; and psychosocial services must be made available to those in need (Rao et al., 2014).

But the guidelines do not take into account the structural barriers women face in actually accessing treatment.

On a brisk morning in Imphal I visit a one-level white building at the back of the Regional Institute of Medical Sciences (RIMS), a major hospital in the western part of the city. This is where Imphal's government-run methadone-maintenance-treatment programme is located.

From the outside, the simple structure looks homely, like it could be used to house the doctors on-site. But as I gradually traipse closer, rows of motorbikes and groups of young men appear.

Here the men—mostly young—file into a narrow, long corridor, one after another. At the end of the corridor a small room opens up to an oversized bottle of orange liquid: methadone. The men write their names down on the sign-in sheet and drink a small dose of the bright fluid. Some stop to chat, others high-five one another and keep walking.

But something is missing: females. Their absence is palpable in a state where almost one-third of injecting drug users are female. And throughout my multiple visits to the centre over a few weeks, I don't spot a single one coming in for treatment.

Thokchom Indira Devi, the regional coordinator of RIMS, tells me that of the 88 clients who are currently on OST at the centre at the time of writing, only three are female.

'Women may be at the forefront of fighting for their rights in Manipur but when it comes to drug taking, they're being left behind,' she says.

Her research assistant, Lolikumar Angom, agrees.

'When you look at the set up here, because of the taboo and stigma, it's very difficult for a woman to come here. The services are man-centric so even though women are welcome here, they ask: what will people think? What will the community think?' he says.

'It's a male-dominated society where men are supported and women are neglected.'

In addition to government facilities, registered NGOs are also allowed to offer treatment. One of these NGOs is Shalom, which was one of the first organisations in India to offer OST. Shalom is located in Churachandpur district in south-west Manipur, surrounded by rolling hills and long narrow valleys.

From Imphal it's about a two-hour drive to reach Churachandpur. In the early morning, a layer of mist hangs over the hills, lifting slowly with the sun.

The headquarters of Churachandpur district is Lamka town, translating in Manipuri to mean the 'place situated at a road junction'.

Shalom is located in an alleyway off the main bazaar in Lamka, otherwise known as the local hotspot for scoring. In the gutters are used needles and empty booze bottles, despite the alcohol ban.

On the first floor of the drop-in-centre is a sparse room that has about a dozen young men lying around on couches. The second level is allocated to counselling rooms and the distribution of OST. The director of Shalom, Puii Pachuau, greets me with a sober face and short jet black hair.

At the time of my visit, Shalom had 200 patients on OST and a long wait list full of men. Only a handful of patients are women, Puii tells me. It's hard to attract women.

'Female drug users are treated differently. Their families don't accept them, so they have to live on the street, and many become sex workers,' she says.

While the space is considered a safe haven, a protected environment for drug users to hang out and receive treatment without fear of retribution, it's easy to understand why women don't want to enter. Like the government-run methadone-maintenance programme in Imphal, Shalom is filled with men. To enter as a woman could be immensely uncomfortable and intimidating and could lead to them being further stigmatised, bullied and ostracised.

'The women often say they feel uneasy to pass through the DIC (drop-in centre) and go for treatment as the males tease them, and even if they did not tease them, they still feel uncomfortable because it is male dominated,' an outreach worker in Manipur told researchers (Kermode et al., 2012).

Another barrier that prevents women accessing OST is the eligibility criteria potential patients must fulfil. To be eligible for RIMS's methadone programme, patients must live within a five-kilometre radius of the centre. But this ends up disproportionately excluding female injecting drug users—many are homeless, like Jenny. Many have been disowned by their families and have no fixed address.

Another criterion for entrance into the programme is that OST must be one's last resort. This means that the injecting drug user must prove that he or she has tried and failed at programmes for drug rehabilitation and drug detoxification.

Drug rehabilitation usually involves medication, counselling and sharing experiences with other drug users. Detoxification is typically an in-patient programme that involves abstinence—quitting drugs cold turkey without any replacement chemical treatment.

There is no shortage of drug rehabilitation and drug detoxification centres in Imphal and Churachandpur, many of which have been around since the 1990s.

Many of these centres, however, are run by the Church and capitalise on the vulnerabilities of drug users to convert them to Christianity.

While the largest ethnic group in Manipur is the Meiti who are predominantly Hindu, there are numerous tribal communities, many of whom converted to Christianity under British Rule in the late nineteenth century. Today more than 40 per cent of Manipur's population is Christian (Office of the Registrar General and Census Commissioner, 2011).

Down a backstreet of Imphal, dense city buildings give way to sprawling land and clean, crisp mountain air. It's here where The Overcomers, a privately-run in-patient drug detoxification programme, is located. The one-level centre has a generously-sized yet sparse backyard with a wooden barn-like structure in the corner. It's a dormitory with beds, mosquito nets and piles of clothes and keepsakes patients have brought with them from home. It's reminiscent of a youth hostel in all its chaos. A few people sit outside and play the guitar, while others sleep curled up on their single beds, sunbeams radiating through the cracks.

The drug detoxification programme is a 12-step programme based on the Bible that lasts for two months. It costs ₹5000 (US$73) per month. When patients arrive, they enter into a programme that believes abstinence is the only way to cure addiction.

The first five to seven days are painfully spent in a small detox room with no contact with the outside world before patients or 'inmates' are moved to the dormitory for their rehabilitation.

'Our vision is to show them the way—that God is powerful and can restore them from their insanity and broken relationships. We don't just treat addiction through Jesus but show that the message can be passed onto family members,' Jterojet Sagolstrem, secretary of The Overcomers, tells me.

The 1990s saw the emergence of residential rehabilitation services for drug users fuelled by the Church's belief that abstinence was the only way to curb this menace. But residents of the Church-sponsored centres were often forced into admission by desperate family members who didn't know what else to do. Once admitted, they were unable to leave and were subjected to a strict schedule of spiritual counselling. Some facilities also used chains (Kermode et al., 2010, p. 244). These human rights violations still occur today in some centres.

In recent years Manipur has witnessed an explosion of privately-run detoxification centres that charge exorbitant fees. Many have been accused of exploiting families' anguish.

At the time of my visit to The Overcomers, there are 62 patients. None are women. Where are the female staff? I wonder. Where would women sleep if there's just one room? How could they afford to enter the programme, especially if they are homeless or without family support? And if women have young children and are single parents, who would look after them?

How can female injecting drug users enter into drug detoxification programmes when they are designed for males, by males and have male staff? In the absence of female-friendly drug rehabilitation and detoxification services, it is difficult to imagine how women can quit drug use and regain control over their lives.

In fact, research has found that female drugs users, 'frequently emphasised the desperate need for women-only and women-friendly drug and alcohol detoxification and rehabilitation centres that are low cost and can accommodate children' (Kermode et al., 2012, p. 6).

It also found that a major barrier for women seeking services, even at NGOs, was that doing so 'could result in the woman being identified as HIV-positive, a drug user or a sex worker (whether or not she was)' (Kermode et al., 2012, p. 6). Being identified as one or more of these perceived negative traits could have devastating consequences.

That women struggle far more than men in accessing treatment for drug use is not surprising given the role gender plays in influencing health outcomes. Gender inequality has a significant impact on how men and women access health services and how the health system responds to their needs. Drug addiction is no exception.

This book has explored the reasons why a girl in India is more likely to be aborted and more likely to be under-nourished; why she is also less likely to access healthcare or to be taken to a hospital when sick compared with boys; and why she is more prone to stigma relating to everything from tuberculosis to drug addiction.

But Manipur is actually considered a beacon of hope, a state which is renowned for leading the way on women's rights. In fact, compared to most other Indian states, a girl born in Manipur is more likely to be educated, to survive childbirth and to work as an adult, just like the women at Ima Keithel, Imphal's market run by women.

But while it may be considered a liberal state, one that not only respect's women's rights but encourages them, its reputation doesn't precede itself when it comes to female injecting drug users.

The previously cited United Nations Office on Drugs and Crime (UNODC) study on female drug users in north-east India—one of the few extensive studies on the issue—found that more than half of the drug users in Manipur sell drugs or sex to survive (Kumar et al., 2015).

Rejected by their families and with few job opportunities, many women have no option but to turn to sex work and drug selling to earn money. Many are thrust into it by their partners who demand they earn money for their drug addiction too.

But both trades are dangerous and fraught with brutal consequences.

✳

It's easy to miss the dark curtain that shrouds the entrance to the Nirvana Foundation's drop-in-centre. Situated across the road from Imphal's main bus stop, the narrow four-story building is a safe haven for female injecting drug users.

In a room on the top floor, as far removed from the realities of the outside world as possible, a group of women lie spread out across mats. They have visited the drop-in-centre to shower, rest, pick up condoms and receive medical care from a doctor who visits three times a week.

Their bloodshot, glassy eyes, their bruised, scarred arms and their tattered clothing give insight into the difficult lives they live on the street.

Jenny, the former school teacher, is here resting with her friends. She stops by every day for a few hours before heading to the derelict house on the outskirts of the city.

One young woman in particular stands out. Despite the warm weather, she's wearing a beanie. The previous night, she tells me, a group of men shaved her head to 'insult her and to embarrass her'.

All of the women I speak with at the drop-in-centre have either been widowed, divorced or shunned by their families, unable to return home. They are homeless and have no option but to engage in sex work to survive.

For the women here, their problems escalate at 4 pm, when the drop-in-centre closes. There is no place they can seek shelter after 4 pm. Some used to share an apartment together but they were kicked out by the landlord because they couldn't afford the rent. Instead, at night the women split into groups of two or three to be safe. Sometimes they take refuge in the public toilets at the bus stop, sometimes they have sex with clients at one of the cheap hotels in the centre of town. At least there they have a bed to rest on. On other nights they may sleep in the nearby forest, huddled together for warmth.

'The big problem is the night time,' Jenny tells me. 'We need a shelter home, a proper place, a safe space.'

The desperate need for shelter for the women who have been evicted by their families or who have no family has been echoed in research which has found that it was one of the things this group of women desired most.

'We need a place to sleep as we drug user[s] are busy hunting for money for our drug use, and most of the time we are not allowed to enter our own house. We need a proper place with food as we cannot sleep in the street, and this will also help us mentally with our trouble in finding a place to sleep,' a female drug user told researchers (Kermode et al., 2012, p. 8).

Consequently, homelessness is a major driver for sex work. And in turn, sex work fuels increased drug use.

Jenny doesn't remember the exact year she began taking drugs. She thinks it was about a decade ago. The 46-year-old had a fulfilling career as a seventh grade school teacher until she was drawn to trying drugs. Her relationship with her husband had reached boiling point and Jenny was tired of the emotional abuse she was enduring on a daily basis.

'He would say bad words, shouting stupid, stupid words. He is the cause of this. He doesn't talk to me anymore,' she says. 'When I started heroin, I forgot all my problems. When he started fighting me I didn't care.'

Jenny hadn't planned on making drug use a prominent part of her life. But when she experienced the numbness heroin afforded her she became hooked.

Her husband eventually left her and her drug use spiraled out of control. She lost her home, her jewellery, everything she owned, to heroin. She then turned to the streets to sell sex and drugs—it was the only way she could survive.

'Sometimes I have 20 customers per night. The more customers we get, the more we inject,' Jenny tells me.

'The customers search for us. It's very easy for them. I sleep with customers at night but there's a lot of problems at night from customers and the police. We are all struggling.'

The problems Jenny is referring to is the threat of emotional and physical violence, including rape.

The previously cited UNODC study on female drug users in the north-east found that almost two-thirds of female injecting drug users had been physically assaulted, at least once or more. The most common perpetrators were non-sex partners, sex partners, police and neighbours (Kumar et al., 2015). More than one-third of respondents have also faced sexual violence, with the main perpetrators being casual sex partners, sex partners and police (Kumar et al., 2015). For women who are engaged with sex work, their risk of physical and sexual violence is far greater, with 83 per cent of women reporting physical violence and 57 per cent reporting sexual abuse (Kumar et al., 2015).

Rare in-depth interviews vividly detail some of the horrific crimes women have been subjected to.

'I have faced many hardships as I need money for No. 4 [heroin]. Male customers invite us and say they will pay the money at the place, and when we go to the place they have lied to us, and they rape us and will not give even 25 paise, and then they will run away,' one female drug user in Manipur told researchers (Kermode et al., 2012, p. 6).

As a project manager at a NGO in Manipur said: 'They (female injecting drug users) are facing a lot of violence. They get caught by some strange men in the hot spots and are having sex forcibly—they don't get any money but get beaten up by these men. Very recently one incident happened where they were caught by some men who inserted a stick inside their private parts. It is very hard to hear about such inhuman behaviour, but it is common among the women who are chronically dependent on drugs and doing sex work. Who will complain to police for their sake? No one complains. If it happened to an ordinary housewife people would come out in support. Community people don't like them' (Kermode et al., 2012, p. 6).

The women hanging out at the drop-in-centre are hesitant to speak about their experiences on the streets at the hands of men, particularly so because the threat of violence lurks directly outside.

Every day male drug users, sex clients and drug sellers linger just a few metres away from the centre's door, waiting for the women to leave when it shuts. Some are brazen enough to enter the female-only space and walk up the stairs only to be screamed at by staff and chased out. Some are waiting to buy drugs off Jenny; others want sex.

What the women really want though is none of that: they want to quit drugs and get off the streets. They want a safe place where they can live.

'I will quit drugs, just tell me where to go. We need a safe place to sleep. We want to stop drugs, yes, but where do we sleep? People don't understand us, that's the main thing,' Jenny says.

✳

HIV has emerged as a major public health issue in Manipur. The first HIV-positive case in the state was reported in 1990 from blood samples drawn from a group of injecting drug users (United Nations Development Programme, n.d., p. 1).

The state now has the highest HIV incidence in India according to the Manipur State AIDS Control Society, a state offshoot of the National AIDS Control Organisation (NACO). It has almost eight per cent of the country's recorded cases despite only having 0.2 per cent of India's population (Manipur State Aids Control Society, n.d.).

Throughout the 1990s, the HIV prevalence among injecting drug users in Manipur skyrocketed to almost 80 per cent (Kermode, 2010, p. 242). While the figure has since declined, it today stands at 28.6 per cent (Kermode et al., 2012, p. 2). Though the epidemic was initially driven by injecting drug use, nowadays sexual transmission is an important contributor to the spread of the disease. Female injecting drug users face a higher risk of HIV and other blood-borne viruses such as hepatitis C compared with their male counterparts because of the huge overlap in drug use and sex work.

It is well-documented that female injecting drug users have riskier sex and more of it due to the need to earn sufficient money to support their drug habit (Kermode et al., 2012, p. 2). They are also sometimes responsible for earning enough money to support their partner's drug use.

Risky sex means unprotected sex. Often women are put in a situation where they do not have the ability to negotiate the use of condoms. Even attempting to negotiate condom use could put them at risk of violence.

As Jenny tells me: 'Clients always want to have sex without condoms.'

Sometimes men also offer more money for condom-less sex (whether they pay extra is a different story) which can be enticing when a woman desperately needs the cash.

'Sometimes I don't use a condom with my clients because they give me extra money for it and I don't really care about others. I am already HIV-positive. If they want to, I don't have any problem not using a condom,' an injecting drug user told researchers (Oinam, 2008, p. 24).

In fact, a study by the Population Council found that fewer than 10 per cent of female drug users who engaged in sex work reported regular condom use (Oinam, 2008, p. 23).

Women could also be more prone to contracting blood-borne diseases because they tend to share needles more often than men.

The previously cited UNODC report found that almost half of female drug users used an old needle for their first injection experience (Kumar et al., 2015). And evidence shows that experience set a dangerous precedent. The Population Council study on female injecting drug users in Manipur found that 96.5 per cent of respondents had shared needles (Oinam, 2008, p. 18). In contrast, 13 per cent of male drug users in Manipur claimed to have shared needles in the last month (Armstrong et al., 2014).

Manipur was the first state in India to endorse a harm reduction approach to drug use in 1996 including needle and syringe programmes. The primary purpose of providing people who inject drugs with access to clean needles and syringes is to prevent the transmission of blood-borne viruses, specifically HIV and hepatitis C. Such programmes are also seen as a critical opportunity to provide counselling services and to encourage clients to enter drug treatment programmes.

Under Manipur's state programme run by NACO injecting drug users are allowed to access a limited number of clean needles and syringes through its Needle Syringe Exchange Programme. A major problem though is that women tend to inject more frequently than the programme appears to accommodate for—and far more often than men.

Jenny tells me she injects three to four times a day. She says her friends do the same. She sometimes buys needles and syringes from the pharmacy when she has enough money. But that extra money is only available when she's had sex with enough clients. The fewer clients she has, the more likely she is to share.

It's a catch-22.

But women appear to not be accessing Needle Syringe Exchange Programmes in the first place. Research shows that up to 40 per cent of women who inject drugs have never picked up a clean needle (Kumar et al., 2015).

Clean needles and syringes are also available at NGOs like Shalom that work on harm reduction. But few organisations cater to the needs of females and they also hand out limited numbers of needles and syringes.

Fear of law enforcement also propels female injecting drug users to make risky injecting decisions. Fear of retribution—of being caught with needles and syringes despite it being legal—can drive women to seek isolated spaces to inject such as river banks, public toilets and cremation grounds where used injecting devices litter the ground.

'I can somehow hide the stuff [heroin] but not the needle and syringe. When the police are in our place, I can't inject so I go to the river bank. I always find a syringe there because people throw them near the river bank. I have to take my daily dose. I have shared [syringes] many times in the past,' a female injecting drug user told researchers (Oinam, 2008, p. 17).

Trepidation of law enforcement is not without justification. The Armed Forces Special Powers Act, the 1958 emergency law under which the armed forces have broad powers, is operational in Manipur.

Tension over the law came to a head in 2004 when a young Manipuri woman was brutally tortured and murdered by troops of the 17th Assam Rifles of the Indian Army. In response, elderly women took to the streets of Imphal to protest naked. They stripped in front of the Assam Rifles headquarters and chanted, 'Indian Army rape us. Come take our flesh'. They demanded the repeal of the Special Powers Act. They were sick of the human rights violations. But more than that, they were sick of gender-based violence that continues unabated across the state.

Locals say the human rights violations committed by law enforcement contributes to drug use in Manipur. But for the women who have already been drawn to drug use, abuse committed by law enforcement only perpetuates the vicious cycle of violence against women.

※

Antiretroviral treatment for HIV is available for free at public health facilities across Manipur.

But female injecting drug users who have tested positive for HIV often struggle to access life-saving drugs. For many women, HIV is just another problem in their lives.

They can delay seeking treatment or forgo treatment altogether for fear of stigma and negative healthcare worker attitudes. They can also avoid treatment because HIV is just another problem they are going to be blamed for, just another problem on top of all the others they face on a daily basis.

But more than that, female injecting drug users are often simply unable to access life-saving drugs because they lack the required identification documents.

Sobhana Sorokhaibam from the Nirvana Foundation explains that when women's relatives find out that they are using drugs, it is common for their families to erase their identity, to pretend they never existed.

'They are human beings without any ID,' she says.

Without any identification to prove who they are, they are unable to access ART from public healthcare facilities.

Already an invisible population, without any identification they become even more vulnerable.

Hepatitis C, a virus that causes inflammation and damage to the liver, has also emerged as a major public health problem in the state. While no widespread prevalence studies on hepatitis have been completed in Manipur, experts estimate that up to 80 per cent of injecting drug users are infected. Spread through the sharing of unclean drug injecting equipment, hepatitis C is far more infectious than HIV. And unlike HIV, it is curable thanks to the development of new drugs.

While the Ministry of Health and Family Welfare recently launched a national programme for the control of viral hepatitis, which includes the provision of free hepatitis C drugs, it's unclear how testing and treatment will reach the most vulnerable—female injecting drug users.

Even the women who are not drug users themselves, but who are affected by diseases commonly associated with drug use, face immense stigma.

One afternoon in Imphal I attended a gathering of widows who had lost their husbands to drugs. There, I met a woman in her forties, who had contracted both hepatitis C and HIV from her husband, an injecting drug user. Her husband died in 2008, leaving the woman to cope with the immense stigma of having diseases associated with drug use. Like the women who are blamed for being unable to control their husbands' sexual appetite and therefore are to blame for their HIV-positive status, drug users' wives are blamed for their husbands' drug use. They become drug users by association.

'The way my in-laws treat me is very different from how they treat everyone else,' she tells me.

'They don't want to eat with me. They have a demeaning attitude towards me.'

The other widows at the gathering report similar harrowing experiences. One of them is Benn Benn, a woman whose husband was also an injecting drug user. He died in 2008 of acute liver cirrhosis, a consequence of having untreated hepatitis C.

'I was so scared about hepatitis C. If I died what will happen to my children?'

∗

Arranging to spend time with former school teacher Jenny is, at times, frustrating.

Late one night she calls me to ask if we could meet the following morning at the Nirvana Foundation's drop-in-centre. I arrive the next day to meet her at 10 am but she's not there. I hang around for a few hours and ask everyone there if they have her mobile number. Jenny doesn't have a mobile though—she had called me from someone else's phone.

She doesn't turn up.

The following morning I see her sitting on the steps of the centre alone. She's peeling a mound of pumpkin seeds, flicking the delicate shells off her skirt onto the ground. She's had a difficult night and appears agitated. Her hair that is usually tied neatly behind her eyes in a low bun is scruffy and out of place. Her wicked sense of humour and contagious laugh is missing this morning.

She gets up off the cold concrete stairs and mumbles to herself. She has to get to work.

Despite the heavy police and armed security force presence, Jenny navigates the streets with ease. Her first stop is across the road at Imphal's main bus station. It's a hub for drug users with nearby alleyways filled with used needles, empty booze bottles and the occasional condom wrapper. Jenny is well-known. As she walks casually up the street, a steady stream of drug users approach her and discreetly swap money for heroin. Some guys on motorbikes pull up, do a quick transaction without even taking off their helmets, and drive on. Within half an hour Jenny has sold all the heroin that was stuffed inside the inner zipper of her handbag. It's time to go back to the dilapidated building on the outskirts of the city.

We catch a micro-bus to the edge of town. Jenny sits on the edge of the bus, clutching the metal railing above her. We make small talk as she gazes towards the rice paddies and rolling hills beyond.

Once at the house, Jenny makes her way to the back room. She sits cross-legged on the floor next to the timber table that is covered in needles, water, heroin and an ashtray. She pulls out her injecting equipment and some heroin. She injects twice. Not long afterwards her eyes roll to the back of her head. She rocks back and forth, her head hanging loose and low. She eventually passes out. No one in the room appears to notice or care.

When she awakens later, it's time to hit the streets back in Imphal. Jenny doesn't know where she'll sleep tonight. Maybe the public toilets at the bus station, maybe with a client in one of the cheap hotels in town. She hates sleeping in the forest, so anything to avoid that situation.

We walk to the nearest major road to ride the micro-bus back into town. On the way Jenny stops to buy an ice-cream, its coldness bringing her temporarily out of her drug-induced haze. She floats the idea of a samosa too but soon forgets that idea as soon as she sees the bus in the distance.

'I really want to quit drug use. I need some treatment. Will you help me?' she asks on the bus. Before I get to a chance to respond, she's fallen back asleep, her soft snores reverberating throughout the bus.

References

Aceijas, C., Friedman, S. R., Cooper, H. L. F., et al. (2006) Estimates of injecting drug users at the national and local level in developing and transitional countries, and gender and age distribution. *BMJ Journals* 82(3): 344. Available at: https://sti.bmj.com/content/82/suppl_3/iii10.long

Armstrong, G., Nuken, A., Medhi, G. K., et al. (2014) Injecting drug use in Manipur and Nagaland, Northeast India: injecting and sexual risk behaviours across age groups. *Harm Reduction Journal* 11(*1*): 27. Available at: https://harmreductionjournal.biomedcentral.com/articles/10.1186/1477-7517-11-27

Cousins, S. (2017) Invisible Women: The unseen plight of Manipur's female drug users. *The Caravan*, 1 September. Available at: https://caravanmagazine.in/reportage/unseen-plight-manipur-female-drug-users

Human Rights Watch (2008) *These Fellows Must Be Eliminated: Relentless Violence and Impunity in Manipur.* Available at: https://www.hrw.org/reports/2008/india0908/index.htm

Kermode, M., Longleng, V., Singh B. C. et al. (2009) Killing time with enjoyment: a qualitative study of initiation into injecting drug use in north-east India.

Kermode, M., Longleng, V., Singh B. C. et al. *Substance Use & Misuse* 44(*8*): 1070–1089. DOI: https://doi.org/10.1080/10826080802486301

Kermode, M., Deutschmann, P., Arunkumar, M. C. et al. (2010) Injecting drug use and HIV in northeast India: Negotiating a public health response in a complex environment. *South Asian History and Culture*, 1(*2*): 239–249. Available at: http://dx.doi.org/10.1080/19472491003592953

Kermode, M., Crofts, N., Kumar, M. S. et al. (2011) Opioid substitution therapy in resource-poor settings. *Bulletin of World Health Organisation*, 89: 243–243. Available at: https://www.who.int/bulletin/volumes/89/4/11-086850/en/

Kermode, M., Songput, C. H., Sono, C. Z., et al. (2012) Meeting the needs of women who use drugs and alcohol in North-east India—a challenge for HIV prevention services. *BMC Public Health* 12(*1*): 825. Available at: https://bmcpublichealth.biomedcentral.com/articles/10.1186/1471-2458-12-825

Kumar, M. S., Oinam, A., Mukherjee, D. et al. (2015) *Women Who Use Drugs in Northeast India.* United Nations Office on Drugs and Crime, Regional Office for South Asia. Available at: https://www.unodc.org/documents/southasia/publications/research-studies/FINAL_REPORT.pdf

Manipur State Aids Control Society n.d. Ministry of Health & Family Welfare, Government of India. Available at: http://manipursacs.nic.in/

Medhi, G. K., Mahanta, J., Adhikary, R., et al. (2011) Spatial distribution and characteristics of injecting drug users (IDU) in five Northeastern states of India. *BMC Public Health* 11:64. Available at: https://bmcpublichealth.biomedcentral.com/articles/10.1186/1471-2458-11-64

Modi's Mann ki Baat: PM talks about drug menace in his radio show (2014) *India Today*, 14 December. Available at: https://www.indiatoday.in/india/story/pm-narendra-modi-mann-ki-baat-radio-show-drug-menace-231102-2014-12-14

National AIDS Control Organisation n.d. *Injecting Drug Use: Strategy Report for NACP IV planning.* Available at: http://www.naco.gov.in/sites/default/files/Strategy%20document%20Injecting%20Drug%20Use_final%20V2.pdf

Oinam, A. (2008) Exploring the links between drug use and sexual vulnerability among young female injecting drug users in Manipur. *Health and Population Innovation Fellowship Programme,* Working Paper No.6. Available at: http://

citeseerx.ist.psu.edu/viewdoc/download;jsessionid=82679E34DDF2DF3E0
7C7DCF0413DD13C?doi=10.1.1.175.8710&rep=rep1&type=pdf

Office of the Registrar General and Census Commissioner (2019) *Census Data 2011*. Ministry of Home Affairs, Government of India. Available at: http://censusindia.gov.in/2011-Common/CensusData2011.html

Rao, R., Agrawal, A. and Ambekar, A. (2014) *Opioid Substitution Therapy under National AIDS Control Programme: Clinical Practice Guidelines for treatment with Buprenorphine.* Department of AIDS Control, Ministry of Health and Family Welfare, Government of India. Available at: http://www.naco.gov.in/sites/default/files/Opiod%20Substitution%20Therapy%20Guideline.pdf

United Nations Development Programme n.d., *Socio-Economic Impact of HIV and AIDS in Manipur.* United Nations. Available at: https://www.undp.org/content/dam/india/docs/socio_eco_impact_of_hiv_aids_in_manipur.pdf

Wherley, S. and Chatterjee, S. (2015) India's growing problem of injecting drug misuse. *BMJ* 350:h397. Available at: https://www.bmj.com/content/350/bmj.h397

Part III

Past Her Peak

CHAPTER 7

Cervical Cancer*
An Ignored Disease

Rajokri could be considered an urbanised village. It's straddled between the financial and technology hub of Gurgaon on the Delhi-Haryana border and south-west Delhi.

Wide bountiful tree-lined streets mark the way to Rajokri. The greenery, the almost jungle-like feeling, is a stark reminder of what neighbourhoods in cities used to be, what they used to look like and feel like.

Rajokri's peacefulness is a welcome reprieve from the bustling metropolis of Gurgaon, one of Delhi's satellite cities, known today more for its stifling pollution and over-population than its entrepreneurial endeavours and flourishing restaurant and bar scene.

Rajokri was once a traditional village, one with unpaved roads, with people who relied on the land and where everyone knew their neighbours. It had the usual sounds of a rural village too—roosters crowing before dawn, just minutes before the glowing red sun would

---

* Part of this chapter has been published previously as Sophie Cousins, Trial and Error: India's complicated history with cervical cancer, *The Caravan*, 1 June 2018. Available at: https://caravanmagazine.in/reportage/india-complicated-history-cervical-cancer

rise; pots and pans clattering; and children running on the reddened earth, their flip-flops slapping the ground.

Today Rajokri has several supermarkets and schools, hole-in-the-wall eateries, three banks, and more than five ATMs. Rajokri, in fact, houses the most expensive farm houses in Delhi. With this fact it quickly becomes clear why the streets are impeccably manicured and why the tall trees are perfectly positioned along the streets. But most of its 20,000-strong population still rely on farming for income and live below the poverty line. They may be nearer to schools and hospitals now, but most still live in the same relative poverty they always have.

Meera lives in a one-room shack a few streets back from Rajokri's main road.

The shed is shared with her husband and five children, though most of her offspring live out of home now. It is raining and the tender earth has turned to slimy, slippery mud. The heavy rain lashes the roof and the sandals that sit outside the entrance to the room.

Meera doesn't know her age—she thinks she is between 35 and 40 years old. For as long as she can remember she's had a mild pain in her lower abdomen. Sometimes the pain gets so bad that she has to bend over to walk. Sometimes the pain radiates to her lower back. And sometimes the pain is so tiring, so completely draining, that she finds it difficult to complete her daily household tasks.

Meera has lost count of the number of times she went to a local doctor who dismissed her pain as a stomach ache and gave her paracetamol. She finds the pain unbearable now without painkillers so she takes a few every day. It doesn't help much but it's better than nothing. At some point she stopped going to the doctor. It was a waste of time.

'No one thought it was anything but a stomach ache,' she tells me.

But in July 2017, things changed for Meera. CAPED, an organisation focused on cancer prevention and awareness in north India, organised a screening camp near Meera's home.

Meera had never heard of cervical cancer before, the only cancer she knew of was leukemia.

She'd had few encounters with the healthcare system. She'd given birth to all but one of her children at home and had rarely sought medical care other than the pharmacist or the local doctor not far from her home.

When someone from CAPED turned up at her home and told her about the screening, Meera explained the symptoms she had been suffering. Those symptoms could be a sign of cervical cancer, she was told.

'I was having all this pain, my body was paining. When CAPED approached me I thought it's better if I just get my body checked,' she tells me, sitting on her double-bed in her home, her husband by her side.

'I thought there's no harm in it. I wasn't aware what was wrong with my body. It was free of cost so I went.'

Meera waited six months for a biopsy to confirm what by then she already believed to be true: she had cervical cancer.

✳

In the last three decades India has experienced rapid social and economic development. Simultaneously, the country has undergone rapid changes in its disease patterns. Thanks to development and public health interventions, India has witnessed huge declines in its communicable disease burden along with its maternal mortality and under-five mortality. That is not to say that these key health challenges no longer exist though—they do, and the number of Indians who die from communicable diseases is still unacceptably high.

However, India has made the epidemiological transition from having the majority of deaths be from maternal and child health and communicable diseases to that of non-communicable diseases (NCDs) such as diabetes, cardiovascular disease and cancer. It now has a dual burden of disease.

Today, nearly 61 per cent of deaths in India are attributable to NCDs which are, in a rapidly changing India, driven by environmental factors, poor diets, physical inactivity, tobacco use, alcohol consumption, stress and failure or inability to obtain preventive health services (World Health Organisation, 2017).

In fact, one in four Indians is at risk of dying from an NCD before they reach the age of 70 (World Health Organisation, 2015).

The transition to this increasing burden of NCDs has placed unprecedented pressure on India's already struggling public healthcare system. The country has had to redefine what primary healthcare looks like while being chronically underfunded, spending one of the world's lowest proportions of its GPP on health. As of now, the country spends just 1.15 per cent of its GDP on health; it has pledged to increase this to 2.5 per cent by 2025 (Dey, 2018).

There are an estimated 1.5 million new cancer cases in India every year (Dhillon et al., 2018). While the National Cancer Registry Programme was established in 1981 to generate data on the magnitude and patterns of cancer, many states still to this day have no cancer registries. Even among those that do, most registries are in urban areas meaning that the true burden of cancer is unknown (Dhillon et al., 2018).

Among women in India, breast, cervical, ovarian and stomach cancer account for more than 70 per cent of cancers (Dhillon et al., 2018).

Breast cancer is the most common cancer in women globally, and the second most common cancer overall, with more than two million cases around the world in 2018 (World Health Organisation, 2018).

In India, breast cancer is the most common cancer among women, accounting for 27 per cent of cancer cases (Dhillon et al., 2018). According to the most recent statistics, breast cancer was the first or second leading cause of cancer deaths among women in 28 Indian states in 2016 (Dhillon et al., 2018).

As a result, every year more than 70,000 Indian women die of breast cancer, more than anywhere else in the world.

Meanwhile, cervical cancer is the fourth most common cancer in women worldwide, with an estimated 570,000 new cases in 2018 (World Health Organisation, 2018). It kills almost half of those it affects—an estimated 275,000 women every year, and India accounts for more than a quarter of these. In fact, like breast cancer, more women in India die from cervical cancer than in any other country, translating to around 70,000 deaths every year (Davies, 2013).

Almost all cases of cervical cancer are caused by HPV, one of the most common sexually transmitted infections (STI) globally, for which there are more than 100 strains. There are several well known risk factors associated with the development of cervical cancer including early age of sexual intercourse, poor genital hygiene, multiple sexual partners, and multiple pregnancies (Sharma et al., 2015).

Up to 80 per cent of people will be infected with at least one genital type of HPV at some point in their lives—most likely as teenagers or young adults—but for most, the virus will be harmless and will resolve without any symptoms spontaneously.

However, there are at least 14 HPV types which can cause cervical cancer in women, in addition to a range of less common cancers, including cancers of the penis, vagina and anus. Persistent infection with two strains of HPV, 16 and 18, are responsible for 70 per cent of all cases of cervical cancer (World Health Organisation, 2018).

But unlike breast cancer, cervical cancer is preventable. So why are so many Indian women dying from a preventable cancer?

✳

Traffic in the southern city of Bengaluru (also known as Bangalore), the capital of Karnataka, is at a standstill like it is on most, if not every, day. Coconut sellers walk from car to car in the grid-lock, enticing passengers and drivers by holding up ice-cold fresh green coconuts. Other street hawkers navigate the traffic selling everything from salty spicy snacks to cooking and cleaning utensils. One seller in particular stands out: he's selling an oversized mop—just one—with its rod towering above the cars waving like the palm trees in the wind.

Coffee simmers away on roadside stove tops, its rich earthy smell lingering in the air. The smell of ghee also loiters as hot plates are heated to make creamy, crispy masala dosas, a popular street food here.

Unlike the heavily polluted, sprawling city of New Delhi, Bengaluru has ocean-blue skies dotted with palm trees. It makes walking on the streets, and even sitting in a car for hours, bearable, without the fear of your lungs choking.

Given its temperate weather and clean air it's understandable why the city of 12 million—but quickly growing—is attracting air pollution migrants from Delhi and Gurgaon, and professionals from across the country. Bengaluru is India's IT capital, home to almost every IT company in India and abroad.

Hennagara is a village about 30 kilometres south of the heart of the city. Construction sites and new high-rise buildings decorate the landscape next to villages with mud-brick homes, outdoor kitchens and endless rows of palm trees.

Just before you turn down the crimson, unpaved road to Hennagara is a majestic Hindu temple, one with intricate carvings and pastel colours. It reminds me of the temples in the southern state of Tamil Nadu—the Dravidian architecture is so striking that photographs could never do them justice.

At the primary health centre in the village, a group of women, young and old, and dressed in brightly coloured saris, from baby pink to egg yolk orange, sit on long wooden benches. Their gold bangles shake as they gossip and laugh. It is perhaps one of the few opportunities they have to get away from the confines of their homes, away from their domestic duties.

The group of women—about 20 in total—have walked from neighbouring villages after hearing about a free cervical cancer screening camp. It's the first time they have heard about cervical cancer, let alone been checked for it.

This a rare opportunity, not just for the women of Hennagara, but Indian women in general.

The screening camp is run by Biocon Foundation, part of the corporate social-responsibility arm of Biocon, a biopharmaceutical company. The Foundation is one of a handful of organisations providing screening for women from poor communities across India.

✳

For decades, screening for HPV via a pap smear every few years and more recently through the introduction in some countries of a five-yearly HPV DNA test has been at the core of cervical cancer prevention across Europe, the United States and Australia. Such robust screening programmes—which allow doctors to detect potentially pre-cancerous and cancerous processes in the cervix—have led to drastic reductions in cervical cancer cases and deaths.

But in many low-income countries, pap smears have been deemed unfeasible because of a lack of trained healthcare workers, logistical challenges, inadequate infrastructure, and their high cost. Instead, another method—visual inspection of the cervix with acetic acid (VIA)—has emerged as a low-cost, effective screening test which requires minimal training. VIA can be performed by village-level healthcare workers.

One of the major advantages of VIA over a pap smear in low-resource settings is the immediate availability of results—that women can get their results before they leave the health facility which means, in theory, they can be connected more easily to diagnostic and treatment services.

India officially launched its first cancer control programme in 1976 but the programme struggled to get off the ground. It languished from a lack of funds, other competing health priorities and the fact that the healthcare system was nowhere near mature enough to offer prevention and treatment services in a systematic way.

It wasn't until late 2016 that the Ministry of Health and Family Welfare (MoHFW) published an operational framework for the country's first national cancer-screening programme (2017). The framework outlines screening for all women aged between 30 and

65 for oral, breast and cervical cancers. Initially set to run in 100 districts, the programme is meant to expand nationwide.

The framework states that village-level health workers will be trained in VIA, as would medical officers and staff nurses at local clinics, and that women would be screened every five years (Ministry of Health and Family Welfare, 2017).

While on paper the screening programme sounds promising, more than two years on from its launch, at the time of writing, it's unclear what progress has been made in the districts. Some public health and reproductive and sexual health experts I contacted have never heard of the programme.

The screening programme also raises some fundamental questions. In a country with a severe shortage of healthcare workers, overworked staff and poor quality care, can healthcare workers really take on yet another duty? Who is going to inform women that they should be screened? And even if screening is available, what is next? What happens to the women who are found to have abnormal cells? The framework says that if women are VIA positive they will be referred to a gynaecologist or lady medical officer 'wherever available' (Ministry of Health and Family Welfare, 2017). But will treatment be available for them? Will it be affordable?

While pap smears have been available in major public hospitals and the private sector since the 1970s, they are prohibitively expensive. In 2006, guidelines developed by the Indian government and WHO advocated the use of the pap smear at the district level but such guidelines did not come to fruition (Department of Health and Family Welfare, 2006). The newer HPV DNA test—which enables doctors to test for the HPV strains that are most likely to cause cervical cancer—is available in India but it too is prohibitively expensive.

The failure of most state governments to provide a robust screening programme for women is reflected in the latest National Family Health Survey which found that in some states as few as four per cent of women have ever undergone cervical cancer screening (Indian Institute for Population Sciences, 2017). It also means that non-government organisations—the few that work on the issue—are left to fill the gap.

Three community health workers dressed in green saris spent days canvassing their villages to gather 20 women to come for cervical cancer screening at Hennagara's primary health centre. By no means are the 20 women the only ones eligible for screening in the surrounding villages but there are major barriers in getting women to come. This includes a lack of knowledge about the disease, a lack of understanding about the concept of preventive medicine, and a lack of support from husbands and mothers-in-law whose permission often must be granted before women can leave the house.

In other words, the biggest challenge is getting women who do not feel ill or who have no symptoms to leave behind their families, household duties or work to come for screening. Women's circumstances do not allow them to prioritise their health.

The situation, however, is no better for unmarried women—a woman's marital status also impacts her ability to access screening when it is available. Because cervical cancer is associated with sexually transmitted infections and because sexual relationships outside of marriage are not culturally accepted in many parts of the country, research has found that some unmarried women turn down an opportunity to be screened for fear of the potential social stigma they would face (Nene et al., 2007).

Laksmi is next in line at the primary health centre in Hennagara to undergo a pap smear. Dressed in a red sari and with freshly oiled hair, she walks cautiously to the doctor's room. At the last minute she turns around and walks out shaking her head.

Mangala, a community health worker, runs after her as she makes a pass for the exit.

'I don't have any problem,' Laksmi says. 'I don't want to do it. I won't do it.'

'You should do this. I've done it before,' Mangala tells her. 'It's good to prevent health problems before they come. You can prevent cancer.'

For Mangala and the other health workers at the centre, Laksmi's reaction isn't a surprise.

For some of the women who are able to come to the centre for screening—women who have overcome the structural barriers that could prevent them from coming—apprehension often takes over. And for some, simply seeing the instrument lying on the bedside tray is enough to turn their apprehension into refusal.

'That happens once they see the instrument,' Mangala tells me. 'They will feel shy. They do not want to show their private parts.'

A core part of any screening programme is education—educating the population about a disease, its risk factors, benefits of screening and treatment options. If there are no awareness campaigns how can anyone be expected to take up screening when they do not understand the benefits or what is being asked of them?

'The lack of high level government efforts to promote organised screening programmes for cervical cancer despite acknowledging the importance of the screening programmes, the future of cervical cancer continues to remain bleak in India,' one researcher wrote (Basu, 2006). 'It is overdue that the government responds to the need of the hour and strengthens information, education and communication efforts on cervical cancer along with providing widespread screening facilities.'

If a woman with cervical cancer is lucky enough to make it to a hospital in time, her prospects for effective treatment of late-stage cancer are poor, especially in rural areas with ill-equipped healthcare. After all, less than 50 per cent of women diagnosed with cervical cancer will survive more than five years (Rathi et al., 2016).

This is exactly why the HPV vaccine is so vital. For girls and women across India it is the best—and often their only—line of defence against this deadly disease.

✳

In 2006, to much excitement, the US Food and Drug Administration (FDA) approved Gardasil, manufactured by Merck, one of the world's largest pharmaceutical companies, as the first vaccine to protect against four types of HPV, including those that are responsible for causing 70 per cent of cervical cancer cases. A year later another HPV vaccine, Cervarix, manufactured by pharmaceutical giant Glaxo Smith Kline, was introduced in the European Union in 2007.

There are now three HPV vaccines on the market including Gardasil 9, a new vaccine approved by the US FDA in 2015, which protects against nine strains of HPV which cause 90 per cent of cervical cancers.

It had been less than thirty years since scientists at the German Cancer Research institute discovered that cervical cancer was associated with infection with HPV. News reverberated around the world that there was a vaccine that could drastically reduce the number of women suffering from a cancer that had a high mortality rate.

But with the excitement of a new vaccine simultaneously came the realisation that not all girls around the world would be given equal opportunity to receive it; a realisation that even with the best intentions, it was likely that those who really needed it would not in fact benefit from this medical breakthrough.

Both Gardasil and Cervarix became available in India's private medical sector by 2008. They are, however, prohibitively expensive— priced between ₹2000 (US$27.90) and ₹3000 (US$41.90) for a single dose, in what is typically a two or three-dose course.

Immediately this game-changing vaccine became out of reach for a large proportion of those who could benefit from it. Its exorbitant price meant that the poor had been priced out of a potentially life-saving vaccine.

'We are aware that another gigantic wall is being constructed in the Third World, to hide the reality of the poor majorities. A wall between the rich and poor is being built, so that poverty does not annoy the powerful and the poor are obliged to die in the silence of history,' theologian Pablo Richard wrote (cited in Farmer, 2004, p. 50).

Another wall has been built in India: one that divides those who can afford the vaccine and those who cannot.

However, in 2009, hope that the vaccine may become available to all girls regardless of their socio-economic status arrived. This hope was hinged on an international study that would 'help the Ministry of Health and Family Welfare ... with future programme planning, if and when a decision is made to introduce [the] HPV vaccine and/or to expand screening and treatment programmes' (PATH, 2010).

In 2009, the Seattle-based non-profit organisation PATH, or Program for Appropriate Technology in Health, launched a $3.6 million 'post licensure demonstration project' involving the HPV vaccine in the western state of Gujarat and the south-eastern state of Andhra Pradesh. The study was funded by the Bill & Melinda Gates Foundation and the organisation worked in collaboration with the two state governments and the Indian Council of Medical Research (ICMR). The study was part of a global project titled 'HPV Vaccine: Evidence for Impact', with similar projects in Uganda, Peru and Vietnam. Its goal, according to PATH, 'was to help countries learn how to reach young girls with the vaccine' and to understand such things as 'what sociocultural barriers may impede acceptance of the vaccine' (PATH, 2006).

In India the study involved vaccinating 13,000 girls aged 10 to 14 in Andhra Pradesh with Gardasil and 10,000 girls with Cervarix in Gujarat. While clinical trials across the globe had previously shown that both vaccines were safe and efficacious (after all, the vaccine was licensed in India), the study aimed to explore appropriate vaccine delivery strategies and provide evidence to the government to enable it to make an informed decision. The study analysed, for example, whether delivering vaccines at schools or healthcare centres would be best. Or would a combination approach be required?

Several months into the study, in March 2010, news broke that seven girls participating in it had died—five in Andhra Pradesh and two in Gujarat. Local media reports, which soon became national headlines, quickly but incorrectly drew a connection between the vaccine and the deaths.

In a letter to Ghulam Nabi Azad, the then-Union Minister for Health and Family Welfare, several activists, prominent public health organisations and medical professionals demanded that 'all trials and studies be brought immediately to a halt' until questions relating to the 'safety, efficacy and cost-effectiveness of the planned intervention' could be answered (Sama et al., 2009).

This wasn't the first time activists and civil society groups had voiced their concerns about the study—some had already raised concerns about a lack of transparency in the conduct of the study.

The government moved quickly to suspend the study and create a committee of inquiry to investigate if there was indeed a link between the deaths and the vaccine, as well as to investigate if there were any ethical issues of subjecting children of marginalised populations to the study.

Many wondered why tribal girls living in rural areas of Gujarat and Andhra Pradesh were selected for the study. Wouldn't girls living in Delhi suffice? Or what about girls in West Bengal? Or the mountains of Himachal Pradesh? If the project's aim was to illustrate appropriate vaccine delivery strategies, then it is only reasonable it would be carried out in diverse settings, including in India's most far-flung areas where the country's most marginalised live. After all, it was these girls who could benefit most from the vaccine.

While little research has been done on the prevalence of HPV among girls and women across large swaths of India, recent research from eight geographically and culturally distinct tribes across Chhattisgarh, Jharkhand and Madhya Pradesh found that almost 13 per cent of girls and women involved in the study aged between nine and 25 were infected with HPV (Sharma et al., 2015). Nearly two-thirds of those infected with HPV were infected with a high-risk subtype—the precise strains that the vaccine prevents. Of major concern is that the prevalence of HPV among these tribal girls and women is four times the prevalence among adolescent girls in the general Indian population (Sharma et al., 2015).

In 2011, the committee appointed by the government to lead the inquiry found there was 'no common pattern to the deaths that would suggest they were caused by the vaccine' (Government of India Committee, 2011, p. 14). Two of the seven girls were found to have committed suicide, one had fallen into a well, one had died from a snake bite and another of malaria. The causes of death for the other two girls were less certain—one possibly died from high fever, and the second from a suspected case of cerebral haemorrhage.

The inquiry report found that other than 'several minor deficiencies,' there was 'no major violation of any ethical norm' (Government of India Committee, 2011, p. 77). The most 'significant deficiency' in the study was its failure to obtain informed consent (Government of India Committee, 2011, p. 70). In the majority of cases, the committee found it was school authorities, and not parents, who had signed off on behalf of the young girls who received the vaccinations. It also found that trial managers had not set up a mechanism for reporting any adverse effects such as pain at the site of injection and in rare cases, severe allergic reactions, and that PATH did not provide for urgent medical attention in case of serious adverse events whether known or unexpected (Government of India Committee, 2011, p. 56). Moreover, it said that because the study 'included vulnerable population[s] special care should have been taken about obtaining of consent' (Government of India Committee, 2011, p. 71).

While the internal inquiry found that the deaths were not related to the vaccine and there was 'no major violation of any ethical norm', two years later in August 2013 the Parliamentary Standing Committee on Health and Family Welfare recommended legal action against PATH, accusing it of violating ethical standards and national law.

In a 59-page report titled 'Alleged Irregularities in the Conduct of Studies using HPV Vaccine' that was presented to the lower house of parliament, the committee said it found 'the entire matter very intriguing and fishy', arguing that the programme's choice of countries and population groups, and the unlimited market potential of the vaccines being pushed pointed to a 'well planned scheme to commercially exploit a situation' (Department-related Parliamentary Standing Committee on Health and Family Welfare, 2013, p. 3). It alleged that the goal of the study was to generate profits for the pharmaceutical industry, which was 'a clear cut violation of the human rights of these girl children and adolescents' (Department-related Parliamentary Standing Committee on Health and Family Welfare,

2013, p.18). It also demanded clarification from the health minister as to why 'permission was given to PATH to conduct such a study on the Indian people and whether the programme was a clinical trial or promotional activity' (Department-related Parliamentary Standing Committee on Health and Family Welfare, 2013, p. 5).

While the Ministry of Health and Family Welfare conceded that that no single event, individual or agency could be held accountable for the ethical violations that took place, it agreed that the study should have fallen under legislation governing clinical trials and should not have been designated an observational study. The Ministry recommended treating the whole incident as a 'learning experience' and that even if PATH stood to benefit from the arrangement, that the vaccine 'has provided a new opportunity for prevention of [cervical] cancer, which is an important health burden for the women of our country' (Government of India Committee, 2011, p. 81).

PATH strongly rejected the Indian parliament's standing committee's findings, stressing that the study was an observational study which involved the use of approved, licensed vaccines, and that poor girls in India should not miss out on a life-saving vaccination that wealthy and middle-class girls in India and beyond have had access to (PATH, 2013). 'India bears a disproportionate share of the burden of cervical cancer deaths, and girls in low-income areas are least likely to have access to the vaccines that could save their lives,' the organisation said in a statement (PATH, 2013). It added that 'it is important to note that the safety of HPV vaccines had already been scientifically established through clinical trials in India and other countries before any use of the vaccines in this demonstration project' (PATH, 2013).

At the time of writing, the case, which will decide whether the licenses for the two vaccines will be revoked in India, is still being contested in the Supreme Court.

As tens of thousands of women continued to die from a preventable cancer and more countries across the world introduced the vaccine into their routine immunisation programmes, in late 2017 discussion around its use in India resurfaced.

In December 2017, the National Technical Advisory Group on Immunisation (NTAGI), the government's highest advisory body on immunisation, held a meeting with representatives from the health ministry, international partners including the United Nations Children's Fund (UNICEF) and independent public health experts. Following the meeting, the NTAGI and its Standing Technical Sub-Committee (STSC) recommended the HPV vaccine be introduced into India's universal immunisation programme.

It stated that the 'safety of these vaccines has been reviewed by multiple medical authorities and regulatory agencies globally', and that 'nearly 270 million doses have been given globally' (Ministry of Health and Family Welfare, 2017, p. 6). In line with WHO recommendations, the NTAGI recommended that girls aged between nine and 14 be vaccinated, prior to becoming sexually active for the best immune response. The goal the NTAGI said was 'to introduce the HPV vaccine country-wide' (Ministry of Health and Family Welfare, 2017, p. 7). The group agreed that the inclusion of specific HPV vaccines in the programme was subject to the outcome of the pending Supreme Court judgement (Ministry of Health and Family Welfare, 2017, p. 10).

The recommendation by the country's highest advisory body on immunisation, however, stoked fire in the controversy again. It starkly divided the medical community, government bodies, activists and NGOs alike.

Rajesh Dikshit, a professor of epidemiology at the Tata Memorial Centre in Mumbai, told the *Indian Express* that the HPV vaccine 'has not been proven to prevent a single cervical cancer death' (Barnagarwala, 2018). 'Let those who can afford it vaccinate themselves. The government should not invest in a vaccine that has no proven results,' he added.

Numerous Indian experts echoed his opinion.

Anyone who believes this fallacy can look to Australia, the first country in the world to roll out the vaccine. Cervical cancer levels have fallen so drastically there that the country is on track to eliminate the disease by 2030. It will be the first country across the globe to do so.

As people peddled their own views about the vaccine, it also emerged that the *Swadeshi Jagran Manch*, an affiliate of the

Rashtriya Swayamsevak Sangh (RSS), a right-wing, Hindu nationalist organisation that is widely regarded as the parent organisation of the ruling party of India had written to Prime Minister Narendra Modi asking him to stop the introduction of the vaccine.

The letter said that introducing the vaccine would be an 'unmitigated tragedy' because 'it is our concern that this programme will divert scarce resources from more worthwhile health initiatives', and that 'its adverse effects will erode confidence in the national immunisation programme and thereby expose children unnecessarily to the risk of more serious vaccine-preventable disease' (Outlook Web Bureau, 2017). The letter recommended 'the strongest action against groups that pervert science, which brings ignominy to the scientific community in the country and sells the country to vested interests' (Outlook Web Bureau, 2017).

Other conservatives cited 'moral reasons' as to why the vaccine should not be introduced.

Why was a vaccine with so much evidence on its safety and efficacy that had been rolled out in countries from Australia to Rwanda creating so much tension? Did it really boil down to the debacle in Andhra Pradesh and Gujarat or was people's anger and frustration about something more sinister?

Following the NTAGI's recommendations, the Ministry of Health and Family Welfare said it would not introduce the vaccine into the country's immunisation programme.

It wasn't just the NTAGI that was encouraging the government to roll out the vaccine—other highly respected advisory groups like the Indian Academy of Paediatrics and the Federation of Obstetric and Gynaecological Societies of India also publicly recommended it. The Indian Council of Medical Research in 2017 also endorsed the introduction of the vaccine following expert group meetings which reviewed global recommendations and evidence.

Yet it was clear that the HPV vaccine had become so politicised and polarising that it was becoming impossible to look at the benefits of it from a public health perspective.

It is impossible to decipher to what extent the PATH study debacle impacted people's perception of the vaccine or rather to what extent people are using it as an excuse to not introduce it. But given that the committee found that the vaccine did not play a role in the death of the seven girls, it is difficult to understand how the vaccine's 'adverse effects will erode confidence in the national immunisation programme' (Outlook Web Bureau, 2017).

One point of contention that divides experts is the vaccine's high cost and the country's competing health priorities.

As mentioned earlier, India, like most of South Asia and sub-Saharan Africa, is now facing a dual burden of disease from communicable diseases such as malaria and TB, and non-communicable diseases such as diabetes and cardiovascular disease.

Some asked why girls should be vaccinated against HPV when children continue to die from other vaccine-preventable diseases.

Many experts wondered: given the number of other health problems plaguing Indians, why should this vaccine be introduced? Why should we prioritise cervical cancer over any other disease, especially when it only affects women?

'States do not think that a vaccine against cervical cancer is a burning need,' Mridu Gupta, chief operations officer of CAPED, the cervical cancer prevention group, tells me.

Others asked whether the vaccine was cost-effective—a rogue term that has unfortunately become a mainstay in public health and the lens through which all potential interventions are viewed and discussed.

But as Paul Farmer highlights, this concept has devastating effects. 'Thus has the notion of cost-effectiveness become one of the chief means by which we manage (and perpetuate) modern inequality,' he writes in *Pathologies of Power* (2004, p. 125).

Interestingly, though, research has found that the financial burden cervical cancer poses over the Indian economy is greater than any other chronic disease with the exception of only cardiovascular disease (Rathi et al., 2016). Just as thought-provoking is that Rwanda—one of the world's poorest countries that suffered a genocide—has considered the vaccine so 'cost-effective' that it has rolled it out to school girls across the country.

Moreover, while India is receiving support from Gavi, the Vaccine Alliance, to vaccinate children against against a wide variety of diseases, the country has begun transitioning away from this support and is expected to fully self-finance all its vaccine programmes by 2021. Gavi, like it is doing in other low-income countries, has offered to assist India in introducing the HPV vaccine, but time is of the essence.

There is fear, however, that at the very heart of this issue is not the safety or efficacy of the vaccine, nor its cost-effectiveness.

'The underlying reason why people do not want the vaccine is the fact it's given to adolescent girls,' Leela Visaria, a social researcher and honorary professor at the Gujarat Institute of Development Research, tells me.

The issue with giving the vaccine to adolescent girls, she says, is that people 'fear that girls will become promiscuous. People take this moral [view point] and ask: how can you introduce something like this for young girls?'

It's a view that has, sadly to the detriment of young girls and women, become very popular.

Unfortunately, though, this increasingly mainstream view is even thwarting efforts to raise awareness about cervical cancer at schools. As one obstetrician and gynaecologist told a local Bangalore newspaper: 'It is a challenge to create awareness about this in schools and colleges because it is often linked to the necessity of sex [education] among school children. In fact, a very famous Christian mission-run school in the city stopped me from giving a talk on awareness on cervical cancer saying: "Our girls are not like that"' (Kamath, 2016).

Research from north India shows that many parents are of the opinion that the HPV vaccine would make sex safe, leading to promiscuity among the younger generation that would ultimately 'tarnish family prestige' (Hussain et al., 2014).

Sanghamitra Singh from the Population Foundation of India says that discussions surrounding the vaccine had failed to focus on the benefits of it.

'The question here is not about promoting sexual activity,' she tells me, 'it's about the efficacy of the vaccine... which is more effective when given to girls before they're sexually active.' She likened the misconception around HPV vaccination to 'educating a young boy about condoms but saying it will encourage him to have sex. It's very bizarre. Prevention is better than cure and that is what the vaccine is trying to do.'

A few states, however, have ignored concerns around the vaccine's 'cost-effectiveness', competing health priorities and the belief that it sexualises girls. In 2016, Delhi and Punjab, and more recently the north-eastern state of Sikkim, began an HPV vaccination programme for school girls aged 11 to 13. It can only be hoped that in time other states follow suit.

✳

It took Meera six months to undergo a biopsy following her positive screening examination performed by CAPED near her home in Delhi.

Every 10 days she made the arduous journey from her home, leaving at 5.30 am, to a hospital in Delhi where she would join a queue and wait patiently for her name to be called.

Time and time again when she would eventually see the doctor, she would be given pain medicine and sent her on her way. 'There is no point coming here. You are just wasting your time,' the doctor told her repeatedly.

Meera's daughter joined her mother on the frequent long trips to the hospital. After months, her frustration turned to anger.

'When you get to know that your family member is not well, you want them treated as soon as possible,' she tells me. 'We were going there every 10 or 15 days and every time we went to the hospital nothing was happening. The doctor was petrified thinking that she (Meera) had cancer so why was there such a hold up?'

Eventually Meera decided to try her luck at a different government hospital. The pair would leave the house before dawn to make the onerous journey, to then join a queue and wait for the doctor who would see patients in a three-hour window.

'By the time my number would be called, the doctor would leave. Then I would wait for the evening doctor but the evening doctor would say, "I am not the one to see you, the morning doctor is the right doctor for you",' Meera says.

After three months of persistence, of going back and forth to the hospital, after having to borrow ₹30,000 (US$418.20) from family and friends, she finally had a biopsy that confirmed what she already knew. The doctor told her she would have to have a partial hysterectomy to remove her cervix. Meera is now anxiously waiting for the doctor to schedule the operation.

But time is of the essence because after all, only one in two women in India with cervical cancer survive longer than five years.

Yet Meera is one of the lucky ones; most women don't seek help until it's too late, if at all.

Meera's case is emblematic of the struggles women face in seeking treatment for a disease like cervical cancer. Fighting this disease is not just about offering vaccination and a robust screening programme, it's also about providing treatment that is affordable, accessible and equitable. It's also about fighting sexual health taboos, combating stigma and raising awareness that women's health is so much more than just reproduction.

In India, other aspects of women's sexual and reproductive health from the right to sex education, to decide whether and when to be sexually active or to have children, and to be free from all forms of violence and coercion, are rarely spoken of.

The sense of shame that is attached to cervical cancer, to even cervical cancer screening, is fuelled by the belief that the disease is a direct consequence of promiscuity. Many women fear that if they test positive for HPV they will be accused of acting immorally, and be ostracised by their family and community.

'Because cervical cancer has to do with your private parts, people think all different things,' Lovnish, a health volunteer who goes out to the villages in Haryana every month to educate women about the disease, tells me at her home.

'There's so much stigma and discrimination.'

The sense of shame associated with the disease among those who are found to have the disease can have devastating consequences. As Mridu Gupta tells me: 'Women who are confirmed to have cervical cancer have a difficult journey. I haven't seen families take women for treatment. It usually gets left.'

Whatever the result of the pending Supreme Court judgement, women's lives hang in the balance. Tens of thousands of women are dying from a cancer that can be prevented through vaccination and a robust screening programme. But as long as the premature deaths of women are not a primary discussion point among policy-makers, deaths will continue and most will happen among the poor—those who cannot afford the vaccine, who lack knowledge of the disease and who face unrelenting structural barriers in accessing healthcare.

At the end of the day, gender inequality may well prove the biggest threat to medical breakthroughs like the HPV vaccine.

References

Barnagarwala, T. (2018) Why the vaccine against cervical cancer is not such a simple shot. *The Indian Express*, 10 January. Available at: https://indianexpress.com/article/explained/why-the-vaccine-against-cervical-cancer-is-not-such-a-simple-shot-4980018/

Basu, M. (2006) The relevance of cervical cancer screening and the future of cervical cancer control in India in the light of the approval of the vaccine against cervical cancer. *Indian Journal of Cancer* 43(3): 139.

Davies, W. (2013) India has most cervical cancer deaths. *The Wall Street Journal*, 10 May. Available at: https://blogs.wsj.com/indiarealtime/2013/05/10/india-has-highest-number-of-cervical-cancer-deaths/

Department of Health and Family Welfare (2006) *National Cancer Control Programme*. Ministry of Health and Family Welfare, Government of India. Available at: https://mohfw.gov.in/about-us/departments/departments-health-and-family-welfare/national-cancer-control-programme

Department-related Parliamentary Standing Committee on Health and Family Welfare (2013) *Alleged Irregularities in the Conduct of Studies using Human Papilloma Virus (HPV) Vaccine by Path in India (Department of Health Research, Ministry of Health and Family Welfare)*. Report for Parliament of India: Rajya Sabha, Report No. 72. Available at: http://164.100.47.5/newcommittee/ reports/EnglishCommittees/Committee%20on%20Health%20and%20 Family%20Welfare/72.pdf

Dey, S. (2018) India to increase public health spending to 2.5% of its GDP. *The Times of India*, 12 December. Available at: https://timesofindia.indiatimes. com/india/india-to-increase-public-health-spending-to-2-5-of-its-gdp-by-2025-pm-modi/articleshow/67064178.cms

Dhillon, P. K., Mathur, P., Nandakumar, A. et al. (2018) The burden of cancers and their variations across the states of India: The global burden of disease study 1990–2016. *The Lancet* 19(*10*): 1289–1306. Available at: https://www.thelancet. com/journals/lanonc/article/PIIS1470-2045(18)30447-9/fulltext#%20

Farmer, P. (2004) *Pathologies of Power: Health, Human Rights, and the New War on the Poor*. California: University of California Press.

Government of India Committee (2011) 'Alleged irregularities in the conduct of studies using Human Papilloma Virus (HPV) vaccine' by PATH in India. Report for Government of India, 15 February. Available at: https://www. icmr.nic.in/sites/default/files/reports/HPV_PATH_final_report.pdf

Hussain, S., Nasare, V., Kumari, M. et al. (2014) Perception of human Papillomavirus infection, cervical cancer and HPV vaccination in North Indian population. *PLoS ONE* 9(*11*): e112861. Available at: https://journals.plos. org/plosone/article/citation?id=10.1371/journal.pone.0112861

International Institute for Population Sciences (2017) *National Family Health Survey*-4 (2015–2016), *India*. Ministry of Health and Family Welfare, Government of India. Available at: http://rchiips.org/nfhs/factsheet_ NFHS-4.shtml

Kamath, V. (2016) Promiscuity fears fail anti-cervical cancer vaccination. *Bangalore Mirror*, 12 March. Available at: https://bangaloremirror.indiatimes.com/ bangalore/others/promiscuity-fears-fail-anti-cervical-cancer-vaccination/ articleshow/51363528.cms

Ministry of Health and Family Welfare (2017) *Minutes of the Meeting of the National Technical Advisory Group on Immunization (NTAGI)*, Government of India. Available at: https://mohfw.gov.in/sites/default/files/Approved%20 Minutes%20of%20NTAGI%20meeting%20held%20on%20December%20 19%202017.pdf

Ministry of Health and Family Welfare (2017) *Operational Framework: Management of Common Cancers*. Government of India. Available at: http://cancerindia.org.in/wp-content/uploads/2017/11/Operational_ Framework_Management_of_Common_Cancers.pdf

Nene, B., Jayant, K., Arrossi, S. et al. (2007) Determinants of women's participation in cervical cancer screening trial, Maharashtra, India. *Bulletin of the World Health Organization* 85(*4*): 245–324. Available at: https://www.who.int/bulletin/volumes/85/4/06-031195/en/

Outlook Web Bureau (2017) RSS-Affiliate Swadeshi Jagran Manch writes to PM Modi not to introduce HPV vaccine. *Outlook India,* 05 December. Available at: https://www.outlookindia.com/website/story/rss-affiliate-swadeshi-jagran-manch-writes-to-pm-modi-not-to-introduce-hpv-vacci/305219

PATH (2007) *Cervical Cancer Vaccine Project.* Available at: http://www.rho.org/files/PATH_CC_vaccine_project_factsheet_update_May_07.pdf

PATH (2010) Update: PATH's HPV vaccine project in India. *PATH,* 27 April. Available at: https://www.path.org/media-center/update-paths-hpv-vaccine-project-in-india/

PATH (2013) Statement from PATH: cervical cancer demonstration project in India. *PATH,* 3 September. Available at: https://path.org/media-center/statement-from-path-cervical-cancer-demonstration-project-in-india/

Rathi, A., Garg, S. and Meena, G. S. (2016) Human Papilloma virus vaccine in Indian Settings: Need of the hour. *Journal of Vaccines and Vaccination* 7(*6*): 346. Available at: https://pdfs.semanticscholar.org/4f0c/cb777a74f6f9ffb4b5201ce07ae802917d67.pdf

Sama et al. (2009), 'Memorandum on concerns around HPV vaccines', *Sama-Resource Group for Women and Health.* Available at: http://www.samawomenshealth.in/memorandum-on-concerns-around-hpv-vaccines

Sharma, K., Kathait, A., Jain, A. et al. (2015) Higher prevalence of human Papilloma virus infection in adolescent and young adult girls belonging to different Indian tribes with varied socio-sexual lifestyle. *PLoS ONE* 10(*5*): e0125693. Available at: https://journals.plos.org/plosone/article/citation?id=10.1371/journal.pone.0125693

World Health Organisation (2015) India: First to adapt the Global Monitoring Framework on noncommunicable diseases (NCDs). Available at: https://www.who.int/features/2015/ncd-india/en/

World Health Organisation (2017) *Noncommunicable Diseases: Progress Monitor 2017.* Available at: https://apps.who.int/iris/bitstream/handle/10665/258940/9789241513029-eng.pdf?sequence=1

World Health Organisation (2018) *Cancer.* Available at: https://www.who.int/news-room/fact-sheets/detail/cancer

CHAPTER 8

Widowed Women
The Toll of Neglect

The train chugs south out of New Delhi's Hazrat Nizamuddin railway station, passing flimsy timber huts with tarpaulin roofs, children running in between the train tracks and mounds of rubbish, piled almost as high as the train itself.

As we move slowly out of Delhi the landscape gradually changes from overcrowded slums to fields of grass as far as the eye can see, weathered trees and rows of mud-brick homes. The changing landscape also brings with it an array of different sounds and smells—the clamouring of pots and pans, chickens squabbling and the smell of onion and garlic cooking away on stove-tops.

There is something so special about train journeys in India—the rare glimpse into people's lives, the spectacular scenery, the characters you have the immense pleasure of meeting on long, winding journeys.

The train is heading towards Agra, home of the majestic Taj Mahal, but before it reaches there it stops at Mathura junction after almost three hours of travelling. Mathura is in Uttar Pradesh, India's most populous state. It's the gateway to Vrindavan, one of India's most holy towns, believed to be the birthplace of Lord Krishna, one of the most revered Gods in Hinduism.

It's located on the banks of the Yamuna, the second largest tributary river of the Ganges. Lord Krishna, according to the Mahabharata, one of the major Sanskrit epics of ancient India, was born in the nearby forest and it was here where he courted the divine Radha and she returned his affections. The two names have ever since been entwined.

Vrindavan is dotted with more than 5000 temples, dozens of ghats and ashrams, and endless rows of souvenir shops selling every type of Lord Krishna keepsake you could imagine from key rings, to posters, to figurines. The town, as one of the most visited pilgrimage sites in India, is filled with thousands of tourists who have flocked here to pay their respects.

But while the town is revered as the birth place of Lord Kirshna, it is also known as the 'City of Widows'. While tourists head in droves to any number of the temples in town, thousands of widows dressed in white line the entrances begging for food, money and shelter.

The town is home to more than 10,000 widows who have either been disowned by their families or who are simply alone in the world.

∗

Seven years ago, 95-year-old Ravi Das travelled 1400 kilometres from her home in Kolkata, the capital of the eastern Indian state of West Bengal, to Vrindavan to begin a new life. She traversed the country on train for more than 24 hours alone, her few belongings in tow.[1]

Ravi has thinning grey hair that she ties in a low bun behind her ears and a wrinkled, sun-drenched face. The lines on her face, which are particularly acute around her eyes, tell a thousand stories—stories of the hardships she has faced in her long life. Despite her old age and the long list of tragedies she has faced, Ravi's memory is sharp and so is her sense of humour.

---

[1] Part of this story has been published previously in Sophie Cousins, SBS, 2018. November 6, SBS. Available at: https://www.sbs.com.au/news/the-town-of-10-000-widows-where-women-are-starting-to-rebel

Ravi grew up with three older brothers—she was the only girl child of her family. Her father died before she was born. She attended school for a few years, but not long enough to become literate before she was married off at the age of 13. Within just a few years she had seven children—five girls and two boys.

'In my family I was neglected because I had three older brothers,' she says, her voice trembling as she speaks.

'Life has been full of sorrow since my childhood.'

Forty-five years ago, Ravi's husband died after a prolonged illness. After her husband became sick, the family lost their only source of income. Ravi had been preoccupied with looking after their children and staying at home carrying out domestic duties. She had rarely left home.

'We saw very bad days when my husband was bed-ridden for two years before he died. We didn't have enough food to eat. My children didn't get enough food. After he died, I had to work. Whatever ornaments I had, after my husband died I sold them off. With that money I was able to take care of my children,' she tells me.

But the money didn't last long. Without an education and without any work experience outside the home, Ravi's work opportunities were limited. She eventually picked up work at a local textile factory and began cooking at people's homes. The hours were long, the pay was bad and she had seven children to look after. Her problems were only compounded by the fact that she was a widow.

'I have faced so many difficulties being a widow,' she says.

'Whenever I die I will get peace. I'm just counting my days.'

✳

This book has documented how gender-based discrimination and stigma affects women's health throughout their life, beginning prior to conception with sex selection and continuing right through the course of their lives. The natural end to this book is old age and widowhood—a time in a woman's life when the consequences of entrenched gender roles are explicitly revealed. It is within this context that this chapter will go slightly beyond the realm of health to reflect on how decades of gender inequality impacts women's well-being later in life, right until death.

Population ageing is often called a silent revolution (Giridhar, Subaiya and Verma, n.d., p. 1). Thanks to declining fertility, increasing survival at older ages thanks to development and medical advancements and decreasing infant mortality, there is a growing global ageing population. As such, it's predicted that the global population of those 60 years and above will increase from about 810 million in 2012 to over two billion by 2050 (Giridhar, Subaiya and Verma, n.d., p. 1). By 2050, for the first time in human history, the population of people over 60 will be larger than the number of children below 15 years.

It is estimated that by 2025 nearly three-quarters of the world's older women will be living in the developing world (Giridhar, Subaiya and Verma, n.d., p. 1). An ageing population coupled with the feminisation of ageing—because women tend to outlive men—will result in large numbers of women without a spouse. This will affect every aspect of women's lives from their economic and emotional wellbeing, to their mental and physical health.

In India, while women may dominate the older people's landscape, it is still not a woman's world. Women who outlive their husbands will not only experience a longer period of ill health, poverty, financial insecurity but also gender-based discriminatory practices, including the harmful traditional and cultural practices that come with widowhood. It is in old age that women experience the full impact of gender inequality, a result of the patriarchal culture in which they have lived their whole lives.

A woman's socio-economic status is rooted in the gendered division of labour which has assumed that a woman's place is in the home. The impact of being confined to the home, to being confined to looking after children and partaking in unpaid domestic work, means that she has had limited employment opportunities, mobility, education, independence and dignity (Giridhar, Subaiya and Verma, n.d., p. 21). Even for the women who have participated in the labour market, most end up in low paid demanding jobs or relegated to part-time work in unorganised sectors—just like Ravi (UN Commission on Women, 1999).

For the women who end up alone, they are left not only economically and socially vulnerable, but vulnerable to the devastating impacts of widowhood. In an increasingly modernised and urbanised India, the once revered and admired older woman—who used to be looked to for advice and wisdom—has been forgotten, fuelled on by present day trials and tribulations.

*

India has an estimated 46 million widows, the largest widow population in the world (The Loomba Foundation, 2017). They make up almost five per cent of the country's population. But despite their huge number, they remain one of the most stigmatised, neglected and marginalised groups in the country.

When a woman's husband dies, while she may be physically alive, she is considered socially dead. A woman is not meant to outlive her husband—she is expected to die before him, or even with him. Her identity is tied to her marital status—she is ultimately invisible and irrelevant without a man.

Dating back as far as the third century BC, widows used to immolate themselves on their husband's funeral pyres in a practice known as Sati. Some did this voluntarily; many more were forced. Other women were forced to take their own lives by a different method shortly after their husband's death. Sati was banned by the British as early as 1829 but the practice continued in some states (Soman, n.d.) A law was passed in 1988 to criminalise the aiding or glorification of the practice after the immolation of Roop Kanwar, an 18-year-old bride in Rajasthan. Today, stories of women immolating themselves after their husband's death occasionally make news headlines but the extent to which this practice continues in far-flung areas of India is unknown.

In parts of India, particularly in the states of Bihar, Jharkhand, Orissa and Gujarat, scores of widows are killed every year after being branded as witches. Witch-hunts are rooted in superstitions and systems built on patriarchy that lay the blame on women for the death of men whether it's from an accident or an illness. More than 2500 women were chased, tortured and killed in such hunts between 2000 and 2016 according to India's National Crime Records Bureau (Ministry of Home Affairs, 2016). However, the real figure is unknown because most states do not list witchcraft as a motive of murder.

But while the horrific Hindu practice of Sati may be banned and some states have introduced legislation against witch-hunting, in many parts of the country widows are bound by strict age-old customs including being barred from participating in festivals and remarrying; forbidden from wearing any colour or jewellery; and being forced to shave their heads. Such rituals are particularly prevalent in West Bengal where some women are even forced to beg for food in their own home. It is no surprise then that widows from West Bengal make up a huge proportion of the widows in the holy city of Vrindavan.

'Urbanisation is taking away a lot of the values India used to have. We used to say that elderly women are a sign of wisdom and that they should be cherished and revered but that doesn't happen so much anymore,' Winnie Singh, executive director of Maitri India, an organisation that provides shelter to widows in Vrindavan, tells me.

'Their stories are the same: their children do not want to take care of them. If their children don't take care of them, they cannot stay at home. Humiliation gets the better of anyone. The stress that they go through, the emotional and mental stress, it plays a [big role] in the decline of their health.'

Rituals aside, many are driven out of their own homes by their children or their husband's relatives who want control of their property and land. Women are then left to fend for themselves, considered a burden on the family they raised. And that is how so many end up here on the banks of the Yumuna river, begging for food, shelter and money.

When Ravi Das arrived in the dusty town of Vrindavan, she followed in the steps of thousands of other widows before her: she went in search of salvation. She begged on the steps of temples, sitting cross-legged on the floor, dressed in all white. Most people ignored her, some gave her a few rupees or some scraps of food, particularly if she sang for them.

The red sindoor on her forehead and in the parting of her hair, one of the signs of marriage, was wiped clean the day her husband died all those years ago. All jewellery except a beaded brown necklace was removed. Not long after arriving in town, Ravi got lucky. She was picked up by a government-run ashram and offered shelter. She secured one of only a few hundred beds that the government provides to widows in Vrindavan. But conditions in the ashram were harsh and Ravi still found herself having to beg for charity outside temples. She wasn't the only one to find the conditions—with dozens to a room and just one meal a day—unforgiving.

In 2012, the Supreme Court of India said the government and its agencies were not doing enough to reduce the suffering of the widows in Vrindavan after a charity, the National Legal Services Authority, filed a public litigation petition to improve the living conditions for the women. The charity told the court that conditions in the government-run ashrams were so shameful that when a widow died and there was not enough money to pay for the funeral rites, her body was chopped into pieces and disposed of.

Ravi doesn't fear death but she knew that she wanted to live out the last of her days in peace.

After two years she managed to find a place at Maitri India, which provides shelter, food and stipends to dozens of widows.

Maitri India is located about a ten minutes' drive from the main road in Vrindavan. The two-storey white building looks out on a picturesque lake, with a horizon dotted with sun-drenched trees, and weathered grass awaiting the monsoon rains.

The ashram has six or seven rooms filled with dozens of beds and several shared bathrooms. The younger widows who are more mobile stay up the flight of stairs, while the older ones like Ravi stay on the ground level.

Every one of the 80 single beds is neatly made and the window sill above each bed is decorated with shrines to Lord Shiva and numerous ornaments that the widows have gathered during their time here.

Ravi shows me slowly to her room and her bed—she has terrible osteoporosis and walks hunched over, occasionally clenching her hips and back. She chuckles that she wasn't given much milk as a child growing up. Ravi has a bed-side cabinet and when she opens it, she reveals a stash of tea, sugar and prized bright orange mangoes. She cackles to herself. She has diabetes and isn't meant to have too much sugar.

She insists that she—only she—make tea and cut open a juicy mango to share. She bends over and makes chai on her own portable stove that is positioned on the floor in front of her bed, stirring heaps of sugar into the pot. Ravi says that she passes her days singing, praying and occasionally visiting nearby temples. The other women gather on one another's beds to gossip, sing and tell stories of their lives. While they come from all across India with different stories of how they ended up at the ashram, they are united by one common thread: without one another, they are alone in the world.

Winnie Singh, from Maitri India, says that family very rarely visit the women. She used to encourage them to make the long journey home to their families on special occasions, but she doesn't anymore.

'Families visit seldom. We tried to encourage them to go home [to visit their families] but we always found that when they came back they looked sadder than what they were before,' she tells me. 'It plays a lot on their minds and it's detrimental to their health. It's very unfortunate when children cannot look after their mothers.

'We've had a lot of cases where we call the daughters and tell them that their mother is dying and she wants to meet with you but they've told us categorically: stop calling us. Women are their worst enemy but sons aren't any better.'

✳

The women at Maitri receive ₹2000 (US$29) per month to cover their basic needs such as food, transport and medical costs.

While there is both a central and state government pension for widows in addition to the distribution of rations, research has found that women have little to no access to government pension schemes or subsidised meal schemes (National Commission for Women, 2010). In fact, only 28 per cent of widows in India are eligible for pensions, and of those, less than 11 per cent actually receive their entitled payments (Basu, 2010).

The numerous women I spoke with at Maitri's ashram have never heard of any government schemes and do not know how to access them. Most are illiterate and without bank accounts, raising questions about how they would access them in the first place.

The widows are served one meal a day and the rest of the time they fend for themselves using the money that Maitri provides them. It's ample money but still, after years of living at the ashram, they are fearful that tomorrow there will be no food, that they will be forgotten.

'They use to take so much food because they didn't think it would be there tomorrow,' Singh says. 'After all these years that fear hasn't gone away. It's instinct for survival.'

This fear—fear that food will no longer be served and fear that they may one day have to pack up their few belongings and leave—is rooted in the lack of financial security they have always experienced.

As a daughter first, and then a mother, and now a widow, the women here have faced unrelenting barriers that have restricted their access to education, employment opportunities and ultimately their independence. It is understandable that in their old age they are reluctant to spend any little bit of money they receive and that they continue, like they always have, to put their health last.

'We take the widow to hospital so they don't have to pay for their transport fare. They are reluctant to spend money on transport. It's an instinct for survival where money plays a major role in their minds. They will probably suffer the pain but not go to the hospital,' Singh says.

✳

In a major survey of 50,000 older people across 330 districts of 26 states and Union Territories in India, more than 85 per cent of respondents said the health status of women is neglected due to gender bias (Agewell Foundation, 2018, p. 21). In rural areas, 88 per cent of elderly respondents said that gender discrimination was responsible for the poor health condition of elderly women (Agewell Foundation, 2018, p. 22). In urban areas, almost 84 per cent of respondents said that elderly women do not get proper healthcare in comparison to their male counterparts (Agewell Foundation, 2018, p. 21).

Such neglect can have devastating consequences. Given that ageing for women is likely to be a highly stigmatising, ostracising and demeaning experience, it is no surprise that this will impact their health outcomes.

Not only has research found that elderly women are far more likely to rate their health as poor compared with elderly men, but it has found that this belief translates to higher levels of chronic illnesses and disability compared with men (Giridhar, Subaiya and Verma, n.d., p. 21).

An analysis of marital status and health-related outcomes among older people in India found that for women, widowhood was a risk factor for reduced cognitive ability, hypertension, having a mental health disorder, and psychological distress (Perkins et al., 2016).

The study found that 'there is no evidence of these associations among men' with 'recent and long-term widowhood predicting worse health for women, but not for men'. It concluded that 'for the most part in India, men's access to resources does not change when they become widowed' (Perkins et al., 2016).

Widows are also at substantially higher risk of dying of malnutrition compared with their married counterparts. Given that Orthodox Hindus believe that both meat and certain vegetables have pulses that stimulate blood and are therefore impure and should not be eaten by widows, it is no surprise that malnutrition deaths are 85 per cent higher among widows than married women (Basu, 2010). Many are also expected to fast several times a month, putting elderly widows' health—which is already precarious—in further danger.

But a woman does not have to wait until she is old or widowed to experience poorer health compared with men, as this book has demonstrated. In chapter two I examined how gendered health seeking behaviour impacts girls' health outcomes. More specifically, I looked at how and why many parents spend more money on their sons compared with daughters when seeking medical care. This phenomenon, as research shows, continues throughout a woman's life.

The previously cited United Nations Population Fund (UNFPA) study found that among older men and women who depend on their children to pay their medical bills, average expenditure for healthcare and hospitalisation is higher for older men compared with older women (Giridhar, Subaiya and Verma, n.d., p. 26).

The study hypothesised that the disparity was partly driven by the propensity of older women visiting less expensive government healthcare facilities and due to less frequent and delayed visits to healthcare facilities. Such findings have been echoed in other studies too. A 2018 study on widows in rural Haryana found that they ignore their health and consider it as 'normal' until they suffer from a serious medical ailment (Bharati and Mahapatro, 2018, p. 7829).

At the time of a health emergency, the study found that it was the family who determined the level of support and care widows received (Bharati and Mahapatro, 2018, p. 7829). To this end, the pattern of healthcare utilisation was a reflection of the structural barriers that prevent widows from seeking care in the first place. Among the women who were interviewed, almost half said the reason why they didn't access medical care was a lack of financial resources (Bharati and Mahapatro, 2018, p. 7636). Given the dependence of widows on their families—primarily their sons—this is a direct reflection of her value in the home.

Income insecurity is a significant source of vulnerability and stress for older women. As women throughout their lives are dependent on their husbands for financial support, losing a partner means that women are then at the behest of their children for care. But given the extraordinary number of widows who are neglected and ultimately thrown out of their homes, negotiating this new support mechanism does not always work out.

✳

Driving along Marine Drive in Mumbai, the thriving capital of Maharashtra, and rain is starting to batter the old yellow and black taxi that I'm travelling in. I turn my head left towards the sea to Chowpatty Beach where hundreds of people are frolicking ankle-deep in the ocean. People start to scramble to collect their belongings and find shelter. What started as a few slow drops of water sliding down the taxi's windows is torrential within seconds, with gusts of strong wind bending palm trees over.

I'm heading to a slum-based day-care centre for elderly people in Jogeshwari West, about an hour's drive from south Mumbai. The route takes me over the picturesque Sea Link Bridge which provides a spectacular view of the expansive Arabian Sea dotted with fishing boats on the horizon.

The day-care centre is run by a local organisation called the Dignity Foundation and the small, narrow two-storey building is located in the middle of a slum. It's estimated that about 60 per cent of Mumbai's 18 million-strong population live in slums. The term slum is used loosely here. While the word conjures up a life of poverty— one without access to clean water or electricity—millions live with the bare essentials but in over-crowded conditions, directly on top of one another, stacked like matchboxes. Land is exorbitant here. Many more live in abject poverty though, their shanty homes overlooking extravagant hotels and homes, the contrast so profound it's sickening.

In the slum where the Dignity Foundation is located, tarpaulin roofs cover ramshackle shacks that are so precarious that they look like they may collapse at any stage, particularly with the constant barrage of rain. Pools of mud and water swallow up the reddened, unpaved roads, presenting a constant danger to people, particularly the elderly.

At the day-care centre dozens of elderly women, many widowed, are sipping chai as they gossip or read the newspaper. Some have mental disabilities and sit alone talking to themselves. Others have physical disabilities and are helped along by the two female staff who work here. Of all the elderly who have gathered, there are only three men. Not long after they finish their tea, their names are called and one by one they make their way carefully up a narrow set of stairs for a yoga and dance session.

They take their place on a mat and for about half an hour they chant, stretch and get into whatever yoga poses they can manage. After yoga, Bollywood music is blasted from a mobile phone. The elderly women who are able get up and dance sway their hips like there's no tomorrow. Others sit on the edge of the room, clapping, singing and bobbing their heads to the beat of the music. One woman takes to clasping everyone's hands together to form a circle. She gets in the middle and gets jiggy with it. She moves her hips and squats low on the floor and starts thrusting. Everyone breaks out in uncontrollable laughter.

The day-care centre is a respite from the hardships the women face at home—whether that is alone or with their children.

'The women have children but the children don't want to take care of them. They want the support of their children—for social reasons, for food, for medical costs and economic reasons. Often the women don't even have enough money for their blood pressure medicine,' one of the women who works at the centre tells me.

'Their whole lives they haven't had time for themselves. They have spent their lives cooking and looking after their children and their husbands. They call us mothers because they are getting love and care from us. We try to understand their problems—the things that they are lacking in life—so we can help to improve their lives.'

A common thread among the elderly women and widows who gather here is neglect and domestic violence. As I sit with the widows, some come forward and pull up their saris to reveal deep dark purple bruises on their legs.

'My husband hits me,' one says as she rolls up her purple sari. Many wobble their heads, an acknowledgement that it too has—or continues—to happen to them.

Another widow of six years comes forward to tell me that her children cast her out, and that she has a lung problem and no one is willing to take her to a doctor.

'It doesn't end,' she says painfully. 'You get married and then have children and it hurts. I have been a widow for six years and my children stopped taking care of me one year ago.'

Elder abuse is a common phenomenon, otherwise known as the 'Curse of Old Age'. The previously cited Agewell Survey of 50,000 elderly people across India found that there is an increasing trend of human rights violations against elderly women by their own family members. 'Due to their physical, psychological, financial and social vulnerability, they become soft targets', the report reads (Agewell Foundation, 2018, p. 32).

The survey found that daughters-in-law, husbands and grandchildren were the main perpetrators of violations against elderly women. Many respondents blamed changing societal norms for the neglect and abuse—the breaking of the joint family system and the increasing popularity of nuclear families. In the face of urbanisation and modernisation, the trend towards leaving behind traditional norms and attitudes means that women's lack of participation in the workforce is considered a burden on the family.

Instead of valuing that a woman has dedicated her life to raising her family and participating in the unpaid domestic workforce, she is considered a burden because gender norms dictated that she be confined to the four walls of her home.

'My old age has become hell due to my daughter-in-law's cruel behaviour towards me,' one widow from Delhi told researchers (Agewell Foundation, 2018, p. 39). 'After [the] demise of my husband I am like a housemaid in my own house, because I am a widow. Being a widow I have no option but to suffer.'

Another widow from the central state of Madhya Pradesh told researchers: 'My family members don't allow me to participate in family matters, because of my old age. During family functions they don't allow me to interact with guests and relatives and [they] keep me busy with household chores' (Agewell Foundation, 2018, p. 39).

The plight of elderly women in India is shocking but there are signs that change is on the horizon.

✻

Poornati Das has square, wide-rimmed glasses that frame her face perfectly. The 70-year-old ties her long grey hair in a low ponytail behind her ears and is wearing a bright orange choli and a pink, red and white sari.

In 2011, Poornati's husband died, and although she continued to live in the house they shared together, as she aged and became frailer, it was too hard to manage alone. Her son and daughter-in-law refused to take her in.

So three months ago she made the long journey from West Bengal to join the dozens of other women who live at Maitri India in Vrindavan.

'Our children don't take care of us because they are so busy in their own lives,' she says.

'I have faced many difficulties being a widow but now we have people here who take care of us.'

Unlike Ravi, Poornati has rejected the rituals and customs that come with being a widow: she refuses to wear white and loves to wear her favourite jewellery.

'I like to wear colours,' she tells me. 'My son told me not to fear, to not only wear white.'

And she's not the only one—many women in her new community have swapped their white saris for colourful ones.

This small bit of rebellion does not mean that their status in society has changed but is perhaps emblematic of a widow's sense of freedom here in Vrindavan.

'The women of Vrindavan are a community unto themselves and to an extent need to be understood in the context of empowerment,' a report on widows in the holy city reads (National Commission for Women, 2010, p. 28).

For the women who are harassed, who are abused and neglected in their homes and broader society, coming to Vrindavan and finding acceptance, can be liberating. Women may arrive here in awful circumstances, with heart-wrenching stories, but many are able to find a sense of peace and freedom where they are able to mingle with other women, to dance, to sing and receive a small stipend for their needs— the first time many have ever been responsible for their own money.

In another sign that traditions are slowly being dismantled, many widows are also beginning to participate in religious festivals, including the annual celebration of Holi, the Hindu festival of colours.

Dr Bindeshwar Pathak, sociologist and founder of Sulabh International, a local organisation that supports Vrindavan widows, is the orchestrator of the colourful rebellion against traditions. In 2013, he began leading widows in the annual celebration of Holi. At first his initiative was met with resistance, particularly from sadhus, but slowly as the years have gone by acceptance has taken shape.

'If a husband dies, the woman loses everything ... she's not even allowed to sing, or dance. I decided it was time to break traditions and encourage widows to celebrate Holi and Diwali,' he says.

'Culture takes time to change. It's slow. It cannot change in a day. But the perception of widows should change. No one should think that widows are inauspicious. They have the right to live, the right to dignity, and the right to human rights.'

But while the movement may be gaining strength each year, there's little sign that the influx of widows to the holy city will abate any time in the near future.

As writer and feminist Suswati Basu says, changing the taboos around widows will only be 'possible if the government enforces education [to] explain their harmful effects' (2010). In other words: widowhood needs to become a priority for the government.

✳

Ravi sits on the edge of her bed, her frail body just managing to hold up her white sari. She opens up a book and shows me photos from the last Holi she celebrated. While she insists on wearing white because 'it doesn't matter at what age you become a widow you have to wear white', she says she was happy to defy traditions and play Holi with the colours of the rainbow.

Despite these small gestures, she knows there's a long way to go for widows in India.

'Nothing has changed for widows. We have our own sorrows. Our children don't take care of us because they are so busy with their lives,' she says.

As I gather my belongings to leave, I ask Ravi if she has any life lessons that she can pass on—if she has any words of wisdom.

She leans forward on her bed, her bare feet dangling mid-air and with a wide smile and a soft croaky voice she says:

'No child, I don't want you to face the difficulties like I faced in my life. Stay well. May you live in happiness and peace. The work and education you are getting now—we didn't get such opportunities. Now we see the importance, the point, of knowing.'

References

Agewell Foundation (2018) Gender discrimination among older women in India. Available at: https://www.agewellfoundation.org/pdf/AGEWELL%20STUDY%20GENDER%20DISCRIMINATION%20AMONG%20OLDER%20WOMEN%20IN%20INDIA.pdf

Basu, S. (2010) India's city of widows. *The Guardian*, 30 June. Available at: https://www.theguardian.com/commentisfree/2010/jun/30/india-city-widows-discrimination

Bharati, K. and Mahapatro, S. R. (2018) Health care and ageing: A study of old widows in rural Haryana. *Jharkhand Journal of Development and Management Studies*, 16(3): 7829–7844.

Giridhar, G., Subaiya, L. and Verma, S. (n.d.) Older women in India: Economic, social and health concerns. United Nations Population Fund. Available at: https://india.unfpa.org/sites/default/files/pub-pdf/ThematicPaper2-Womenandageing.pdf

Ministry of Home Affairs (2016). National Crime Records Bureau, Government of India. Available at: http://ncrb.gov.in/

National Commission for Women (2010) Study on widows at Vrindavan. Available at: http://ncw.nic.in/sites/default/files/WidowsAtVrindavanReport.pdf

Perkins, J. M., Lee, H. Y., James, K. S. et al. (2016) Marital status, widowhood duration, gender and health outcomes: a cross-sectional study among older adults in India. *BMC Public Health*, 16:1032. DOI: 10.1186/s12889-016-3682-9.

Soman, P. (n.d.) Raja Ram Mohan Roy and the abolition of sati system in India. *International Journal of Humanities, Art and Social Studies*, Vol 1(2): 75. Available at: https://airccse.com/ijhas/papers/1216ijhas08.pdf

The Loomba Foundation (2017) The Loomba Foundation distributes sewing machines to 500 widows in Mathura on International Widows Day. Available at: http://www.theloombafoundation.org/pr/the-loomba-foundation-distributes-sewing-machines-to-500-widows-in-mathura-on-international-widows-day

United Nations (1999) Commission on the Status of Women, 43rd Session, March 1999.

About the Author

Sophie Cousins is an award-winning writer and journalist. Her work focuses on the systems that exacerbate gender inequality and the impact this has on women's and girls' health. She is the recipient of numerous grants and fellowships from organisations including the United Nations Foundation and the South Asian Journalists' Association. In 2017, she was awarded a grant by the South Asian Journalists Association to report on abortion in Sri Lanka. In 2018, she was part of the Fuller Project's Global Women's Issue Team reporting on sterilisation in India, and in early 2019 she was commended for her reporting on sexual health at the British Medical Journalists' Association awards. She writes frequently for publications including the *Guardian*, *New York Times, Foreign Policy*, the *London Review of Books*, the *Lancet, Mosaic*, the *Caravan*, and the *British Medical Journal*. She also consults for the World Health Organisation. She has reported from more than 20 countries in Central and South America, Asia, Europe, Middle East and Africa.